Disclaimer: This book is for educational purposes only and should not be considered a substitute for proper training. It is sold with the understanding that the author and publisher are not engaged in rendering medical or other professional services. If medical advice or other expert assistance is required, the services of an appropriate professional should be sought. Information in this book should not be used to diagnose, treat, or prescribe. The author and publisher shall not be liable for any damages in connection with, or arising out of anyone's interpretation or application of the information in this book. The practitioner is encouraged to always use sound clinical judgment in making decisions about her ability to help each individual and to refer to a qualified professional when the need arises.

Photographs by Brian Birzer
Cover design by Wendy Irwin
Deepest thanks to Tracy Firsching, LMT for her valuable mentoring and contributions to this book.

Additional copies of this book and other books and DVD's may be obtained from:
www.massagepublications.com

MASSAGE PUBLICATIONS
8400 Jamestown Dr #118
Austin, TX 78758
(512) 833-0179
info@massagepublications.com
Schools and distributors call or email for pricing.

Books, DVD's and other products available at:
www.massagepublications.com

©2017 Peggy Lamb/Massage Publications. All rights reserved. No part of this publication may be reproduced in any form (including photocopying or storing in any medium by electronic means) without the express written permission of the author.

Contents

INTRODUCTION 1

THE PELVIC GIRDLE 3

ASSESSMENT TESTS 17

MUSCLE ENERGY TECHNIQUES/CORRECTIONS 31

PRINCIPLES OF MUSCLE SWIMMING 41

TECHNIQUES AND PROTOCOLS:

    GLUTS AND DEEP EXTERNAL ROTATORS 46

    QUADRATUS LUMBORUM 50

    MULTIFIDUS 55

    HAMSTRINGS 58

CHECK LIST 61

REFERENCES AND SUGGESTED READING 62

INDEX 64

A Short Introduction

For many years I felt overwhelmed and insecure about the plethora of assessment test out there. I have thousands of hours of advanced training in massage and bodywork but few of those trainings emphasized assessment tests. Or, it's possible I avoided such trainings because I thought they would be boring!

About 15 years ago I took an amazing class in lower back and pelvic girdle assessment tests and muscle energy technique corrections taught by a local occupational therapist /massage therapist. The class was extremely complex, detailed and challenging. It took a lot of practice for me to feel confident about performing these tests and corrections but I was determined to take my skills to the next level and revitalize my practice.

As amazing and brilliant as the system I learned was, the sheer number of tests and corrections that I was supposed to perform on clients was unwieldy. I sought the advice of an extremely skilled bodyworker who had taken the same workshop. We talked about simplification —selecting tests and corrections that gave the most information and were most relevant to the common problems clients report. Thus, *Stabilizing the Core and the SI Joint* was born; six core assessment tests and five corrections that could be easily incorporated into a session. Other assessment test could be done when needed, such as the Apley Scratch test for the shoulder or the Fair test for piriformis syndrome. Since any core misalignment affects the whole body these six assessment tests should be a staple of any practice.

Using these easy assessment tests and corrections completely changed my practice. I do them on everyone, whether they are coming for chronic neck pain, low back pain, hip pain, rotator cuff/shoulder issues. Let me give you an example of a client I worked with recently:

Kay: an active swimmer who came in with limited neck rotation to both sides; worse on the right. It especially hurt when she rotated right and forward flexed her neck. Pain was centered in mid-thoracic region. She had been to other therapists who concentrated the work on neck and shoulders. The issue would resolve temporarily (a few hours). I performed all the assessment tests in this book and discovered she had a right anteriorly rotated innominate. By correcting this core misalignment we were able to begin the "unwinding process" and get her back to her beloved swimming in three sessions.

You may find, as I did, that grasping the biomechanics is the hardest part of this course. Not to worry, that will come in time.

These techniques will enable you to get excellent results for your clients with a myriad of chronic issues because misalignments of the pelvic girdle impact the entire body.

I've included Muscle Swimming neuromuscular therapy techniques for the quadratus lumborum, gluteus maximus, piriformis, hamstrings and multifidus because of their important role in stabilization of the pelvic girdle and SI joint. I'm not suggesting that these are the only myofascial structures to address – not by a long shot – but they are a good place to start. I also wanted to keep this book at a digestible length!

I want to touch you through this book so that you can touch people and help them feel like a million bucks!

As we strive to increase our technical expertise let's keep in mind the wise words of Rachel Remen, MD: *"We do not bless with our expertise, we bless with our bare hands."*

Blessings

The Pelvic Girdle

Sacrum · Coccyx · Ilium · Acetabulum · Pubis · Ischium · Pubis Symphysis

The Pelvic Girdle

The pelvic girdle or pelvis is the base of the torso and the foundation of the abdomen. It links the lower limbs to the vertebral column thereby supporting the entire body seated, standing or in movement.

The pelvis is one of the key structural components of upright posture; imbalances can have an extensive impact throughout the body. As the body looses structural stability it depends more and more on muscles to provide that support to compensate for the body's inability to meet the demands of gravity.

In successful posture, gravitational forces concentrate at a point where the pull on the body is equal on all sides. This is referred to as the center of gravity, Dan Tian center, hara or core. This center is just anterior to the second sacral segment and is the point where forces from head down and feet up intersect.

The pelvic bowl contains many vital organs including bladder, colon, prostate and uterus. The enervation of these organs comes via the spinal column and through the sacrum. Misalignment, nerve compression, muscular spasm or imbalances in the pelvis can impact the vitality and health of these organs.

The pelvic region and sacrum in particular is significant for its high concentration of parasympathetic nerve ganglia associated with visceral function responsible for countering the sympathetic nervous system (and flight or flight responses), deep relaxation and primitive biological responses to trauma.

In the many millennium old Vedic knowledge base of the East, the pelvis is the seat of our dormant potential or life force and the home of the first and second chakras that govern our sense of safety and stability, unconscious urges and creativity.

The pelvis is the transition point for the single weight bearing spinal column to the stilt-like bilateral lower extremities. If that transition is impaired, our connection with the earth may feel like a struggle. Our ability to be and feel grounded is compromised. This is both figurative and literal as it takes more work to keep an imbalanced structure upright.

The act of walking is one of falling from side to side. A misalignment in the pelvis may result in functional leg length difference making each step a struggle to regain neutral. Each step as we move through life may be accompanied by pain as spasming muscles try to enforce stability.

Even stationary postures ultimately constitute movement. For example, both sitting and standing involve postural stabilization and motion as each segment of the body finds equilibrium with gravity.

Our posture and alignment is a dynamic interplay of many forces, constantly shifting and responding to the demands of our internal and external environments. Our goal in this class is to offer you new tools to restore a stable base, empowering your clients to move with vigor and vitality.

CORE STABILITY

- *Optimal alignment of the bones of the pelvic girdle*
- *Optimal alignment of the pelvis and spine*
- *Optimal movement relationships of pelvis, spine and extremities*

The key to core stability is, you guessed it, the pelvis!

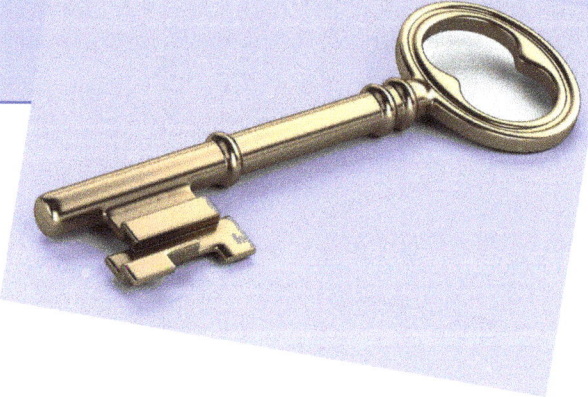

Pelvic Girdle Anatomy

The pelvic girdle is a ring-like structure that connects the axial skeleton to the lower limbs. It consists of the two hip bones (also known as innominates or ilia bones), the sacrum, a triangular bone comprised of five fused sacral vertebra, and the coccyx. There are four articulations within the pelvis all with limited range of movement:

Sacroiliac Joints – Between the ilium of the hip bones and the sacrum
Pubic symphysis – Between the pubis bodies of the two hip bones.
Sacrococcygeal symphysis – Between the sacrum and the coccyx.

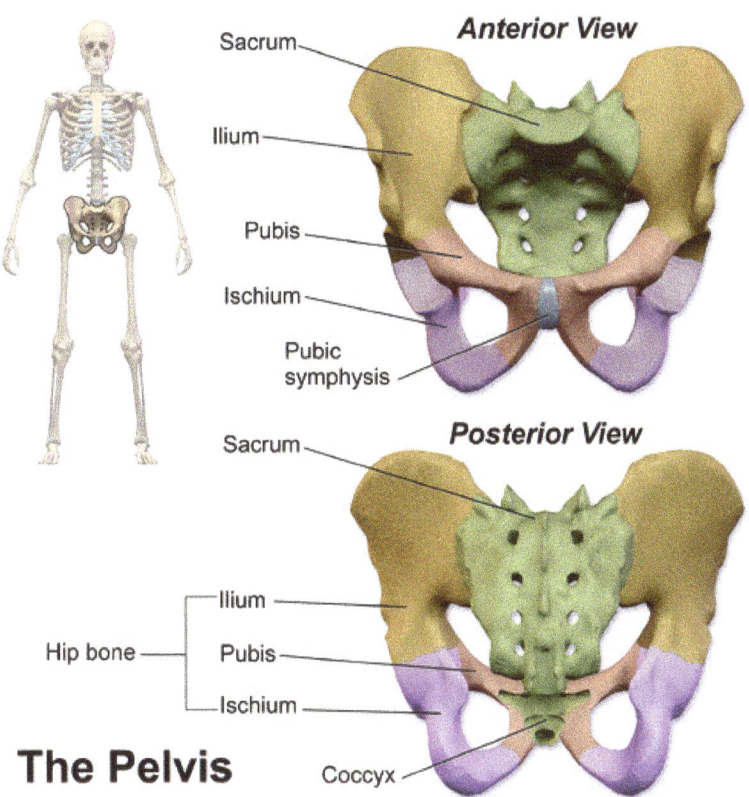

The Pelvis

In this course we study how the misalignments of the ilia and the sacrum can impact the entire body.

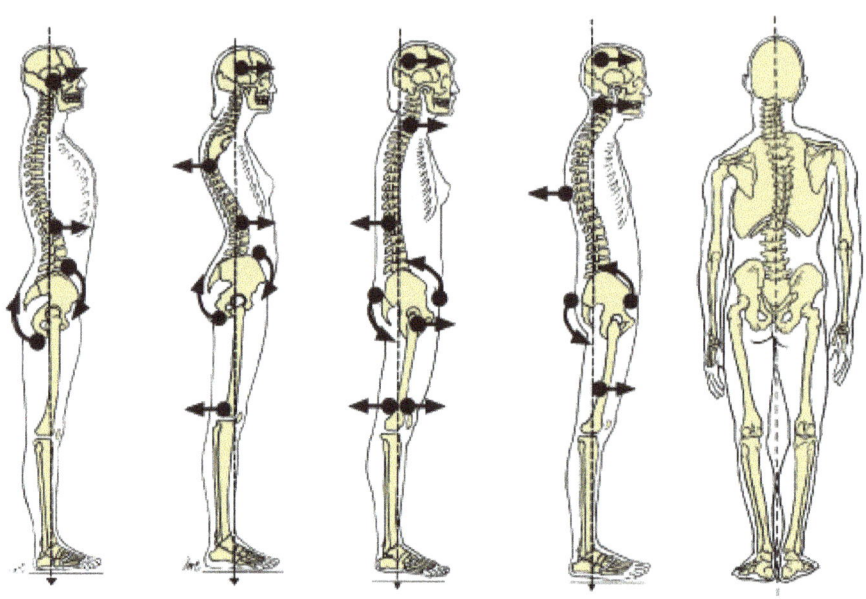

The pelvic girdle resembles a funnel with the broad opening facing upwards while the sacrum has been described as a "glorified wedge" due to its shape and how it locks into the ilia to transfer weight from the torso laterally to the legs and vice versa.

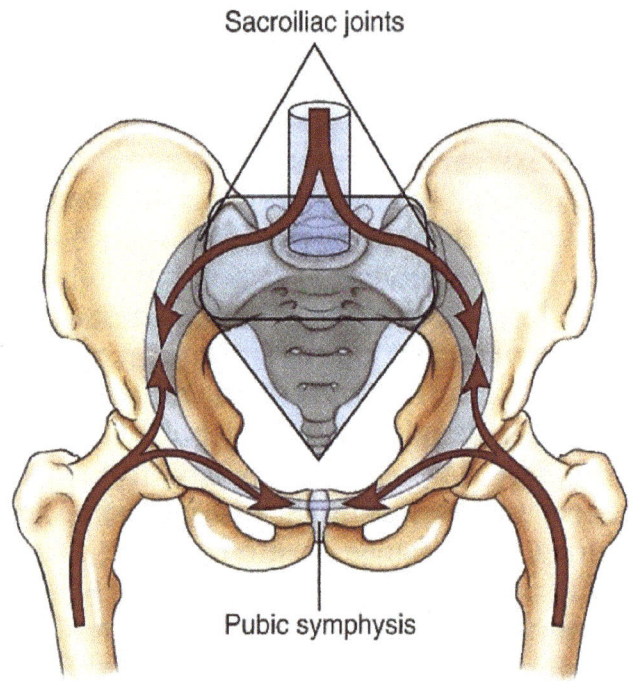

Gender Difference

The pelvic girdle differs between males and females. When comparing the two, the female pelvis (Gynecoid) is much wider and more flared. Using the funnel analogy, it is a much broader funnel. It is also shorter than the male pelvis (Android) with a wide inlet to accommodate childbirth. In fact, all the differences between male and female pelvic anatomy are related to gestation and labor.

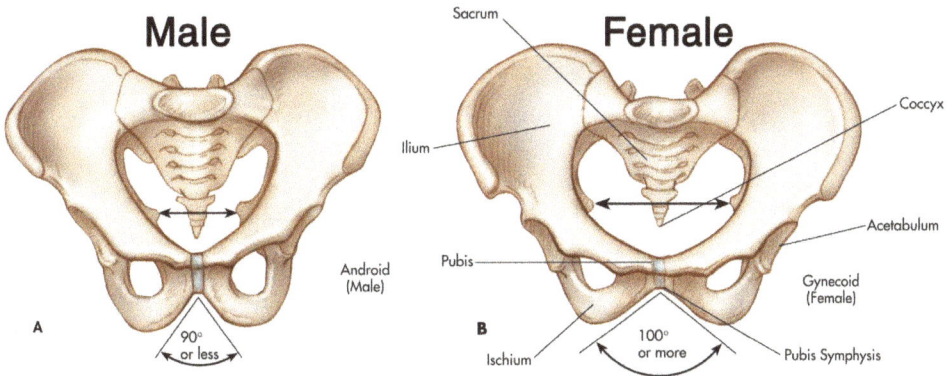

A good visual is the difference between a martini glass versus a margarita glass. They roughly resemble the openings to the male and female pelvis, respectively.

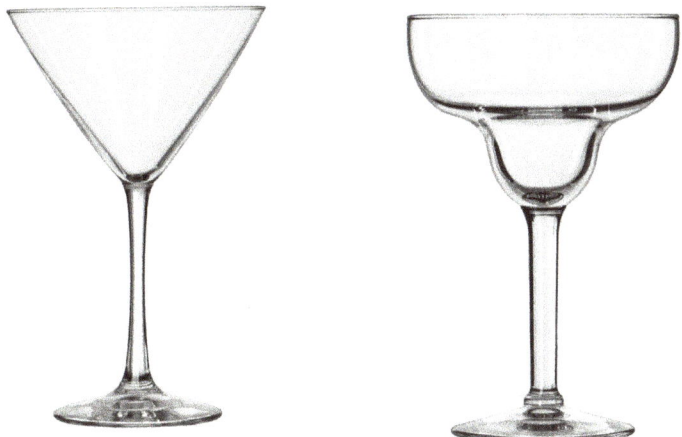

During pregnancy relaxin and progesterone are produced. They break down the collagen in the pelvic joints and soften ligaments in preparation for child birth. Relaxin also spikes in relations to the menstrual cycle. Due to these hormonal fluctuations and the less stable structure of the female pelvis, misalignment of the pubic bones at the pubic symphysis or SI joint instability may result. In other words, the female pelvis is inherently less stable and prone to misalignment issues.

Adaptation

We are all familiar with the cervical and lumbar concave curvatures and the thoracic and sacral convex curvatures of the spine. In addition, all of the vertebrae, shoulders and hips can rotate. These curvatures and rotations perpetually offset each other to keep the eyes level to the horizon. Whenever there is a pelvic misalignment, there is a corresponding response in the spine (often a coupled movement of side-bending and contralateral rotation of the vertebral body).Certainly this was an adaptation to aid in survival. It remains an automatic response and we can get a sense of these complex adaptations with the following exercise.

Standing One Leg Exercise

1. Place a piece of cardboard (a drivers license works too) between your teeth. Your goal is to keep the cardboard level and your eyes on the horizon.

2. Lift one foot off the floor.

3. Notice all the shifts and adjustments that happen throughout the body to keep the cardboard level.

4. Level that hip and again take note of the shifts and adjustments up and down the kinetic chain.

5. Repeat on the other side.

6. Try it with closed eyes! Subtracting our visual sense really increases proprioception.

When these adaptations become long term they can present as kyphosis, lordosis, scoliosis, uneven shoulders, head tilts or dowagers hump.

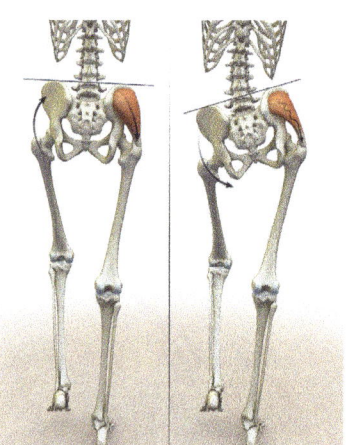

The Sacrum

The sacrum is suspended between the two ilia by the posterior sacral ligaments. Symmetrical tension in these ligaments is key to core stability. Anterior mobility combined with posterior stability provides the pelvic girdle with an effective suspension system capable of an efficient force distribution.

Sacral Movement: Nutation and Counter-nutation

Nutation refers to the superior end (the sacral base) of the sacrum rocking anterior and slightly inferior. Counter-nutation is the return to neutral with the upper promontory rocking posterior and superior. Imagine the big bony top of the sacrum nodding forward and backward. Research has shown that nutation is the optimal position of the sacrum for pelvic girdle stability.

Bilateral nutation and counter-nutation occurs during trunk flexion and extension. Unilateral movement of the sacrum occurs with flexion and extension of the hip joint and lower limbs such as during the walking/gait cycle.

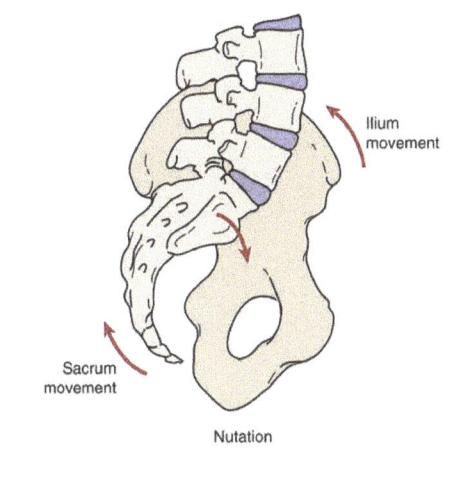
Nutation

Whenever we walk, the leg in extension goes into sacral nutation. As that leg moves into the forward in the sagittal plane (flexion) counter-nutation takes place. We are nutating and counter-nutating as we walk. This also happens very slightly with muscular-bracing nutation as we stand. Therefore, minute movement takes place between the sacrum and the ilium any time the trunk is flexed or extended.

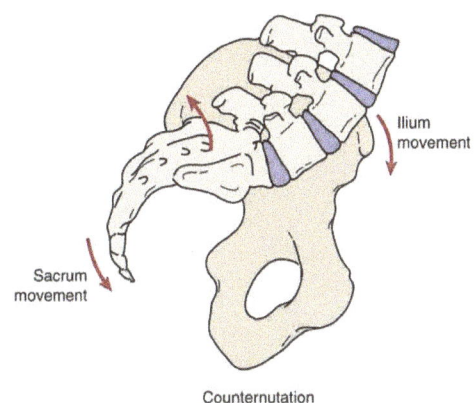
Counternutation

In other words, when one leg swings back (extension), the top of the sacral base nods anteriorly (nutates). Simultaneously, sacral ligament tension increases on that side due to contraction of the hamstring and gluteus maximus. This prepares the SIJ for heel strike and weight bearing. The ipsilateral gluteus maximus and bicep femoris also contract during weight bearing to compress and stabilize SIJ. As the leg swings forward, counter-nutation occurs and gluteus maximus and bicep femoris relax.

Sacral Torsion

Think back to the walking cycle. When the right leg is in extension, the right sacral base is in nutation and the left sacral base is in counter-nutation. You might ask how is it possible that one side of the sacrum is in nutation and the other side is in counter-nutation? It's possible because during walking the sacrum is not in "pure" nutation and counter-nutation. It's rotating around an oblique axis with a little side-bending thrown in for good measure.

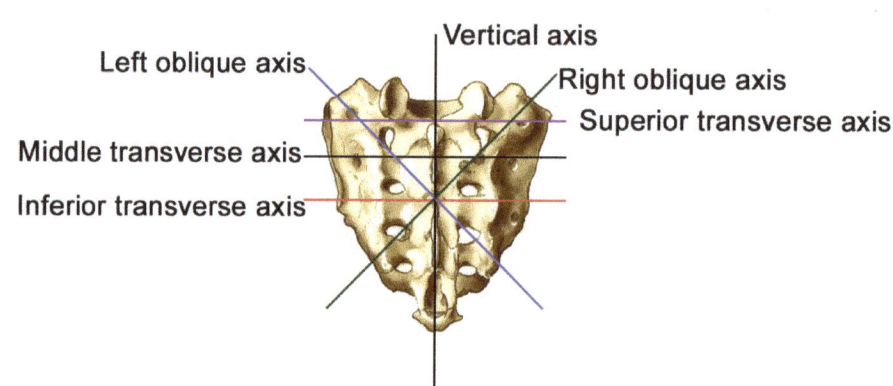

This brings us to the complicated and often confusing subject of sacral torsions. For our purposes we'll concentrate on the most common form of sacral torsions: Right on Right rotation on a right oblique axis (R-on-R) and Left on Left rotation on a left oblique axis (L-on-L). These two movements are natural physiological motions that the sacrum is capable of. When the term sacral torsion is used it can mean either the naturally occurring motion of the sacrum that happens, for example during the gait cycle; or a fixation of the sacrum in this position. A test for a sacral torsion is included in this text.

Right on Right (R-on-R) sacral torsion

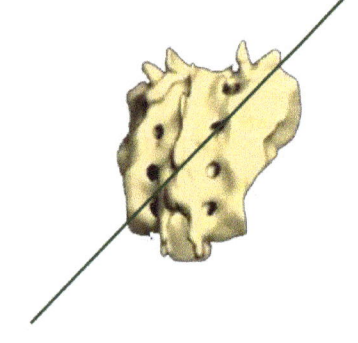

Left on Left (L-on-L) sacral torsion

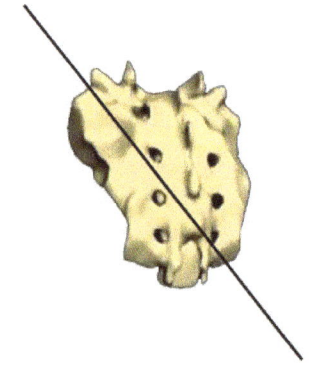

The SI Joint

Each SI joint is comprised of irregular, articulating bony surfaces on the sacrum and ilium. They fit together like mirror images of a 3D puzzle. This provides stability, strength and restricts movement so that the considerable weight of the spinal column can transfer to the lower body. It also acts as a shock absorber. These surfaces lock into place during the push-off phase during walking to increase joint stability. The SIJ only slides 2-4mm and rotates 1-2 degrees via ligament stretching during weight bearing and forward bending. Movements are a combination of sliding, tilting and rotation. Although normal SIJ movement is small, it is essential for normal pain-free low back and pelvis function. The SIJ is classified as a true synovial arthodial joint as it contains a joint capsule, synovial fluid, articulate cartilage and a synovial membrane. A loss of this movement is common in people with low back and pelvic pain. It's been estimated that twenty-five percent of low back and pelvic pain involves SIJ dysfunction.

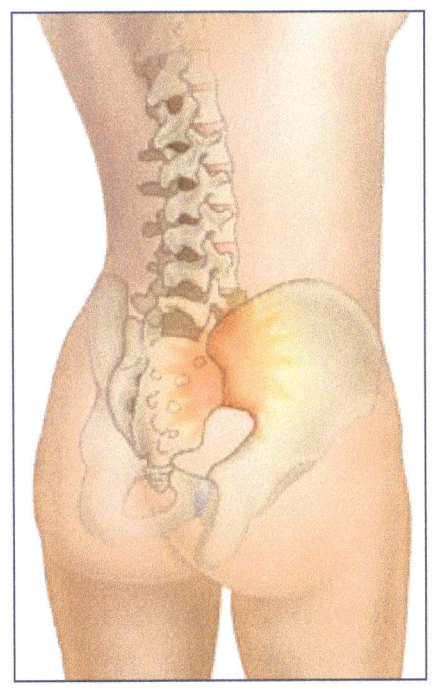
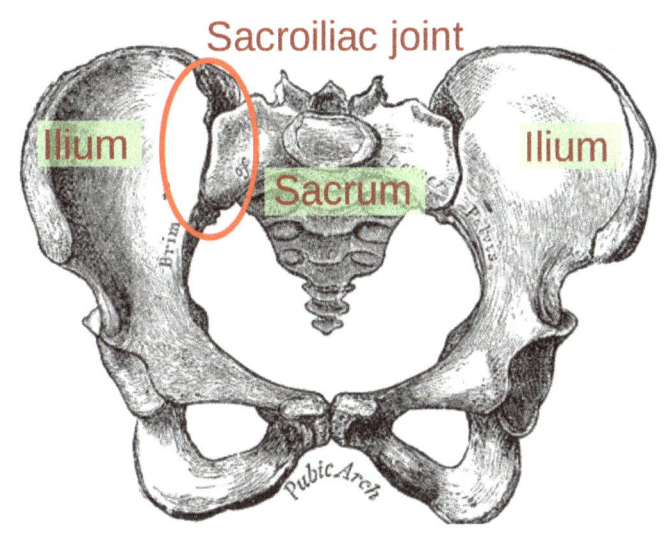

The articulating surface on the iliac bone is crescent shaped and has an irregular surface with a raised ridge running through the center of the crescent and two furrows on either side. The articulating surface of the sacrum corresponds in shape and surface contours to the ilium with a central curved furrow with raised crests on either side.

Self-locking mechanisms of the SI joint

There are two forces that help to "lock" the SIJ: Form closure and force closure. Form closure relates to the form of the bones and how they cleverly fit together to create stability. Force closure is stabilization that results from myofascial contraction. Force closure is created from muscles increasing tension on the ligaments. It's an additional system generated by the contractive action of core myofascial units and slings. When the sacrum rocks forward into nutation, the ligaments around the SIJ and the muscles provide greater stability by force closure pulling the SIJ together. They also increase FORM closure by increasing tension on the ligaments.

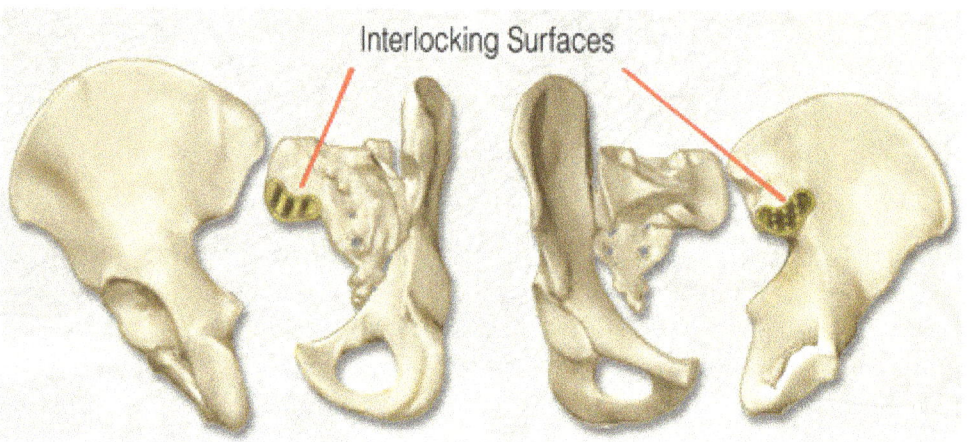

FORM closure

The FORCE closure units of the outer core consist of four myofascial sling systems:
1. Posterior (deep) longitudinal sling: Peroneus longus, biceps femoris, sacrotuberous ligament, contralateral erector spinae.
2. Lateral sling: Gluteus medius and minimus, adductors, contralateral quadratus lumborum
3. Anterior oblique sling: Adductors, internal obliques, contralateral external obliques
4. Posterior oblique sling: gluteus maximus, contralateral thoracolumbar fascia, contralateral latissimus dorsi

Ligaments and the SIJ

1. Sarotuberous: Attaches the PSIS and posterior sacroiliac ligament to the ischial tuberosity. Four muscles attach to the sacrotuberous ligament and contribute to SIJ stability: GMax, biceps femoris, multifidi, piriformis. It resists nutation (nodding) of the sacrum and prevents posterior rotation of the innominate bone

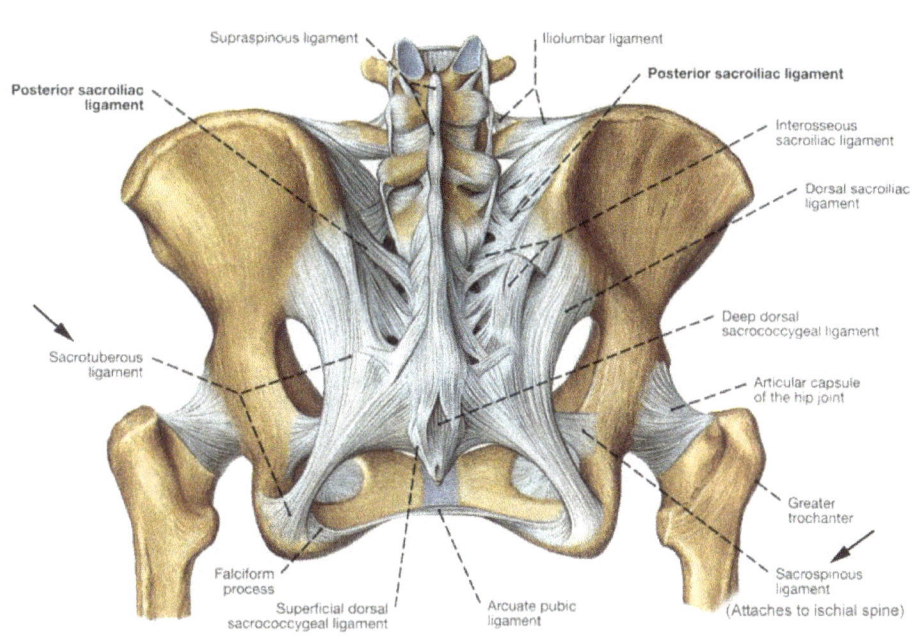

(in relationship to the sacrum.) Laxity can result in posterior rotation of the innominate and increased nutation of the sacrum. **Function**: **Key ligament in SIJ stabilization.**

2. Sacrospinous: Attaches the lateral aspect of the sacrum and coccyx to the spine of the ischium. **Function** is similar to sacrotuberous ligament.

3. Interosseous: A dense, short and thick collection of strong collagenous fibers that attach to the sacral tuberosities and the ilium. **Function**: prevents separation of the SIJ strongly binding the sacrum to the ilium.

4. Posterior sacroiliac ligament (long dorsal ligament): attaches the medial and lateral crest of the sacrum to the PSIS. There is also a connection of this ligament to the thoracolumbar fascia, the multifidi and erector spinae muscles. **Function**: resists counter-nutation of the sacrum. If sacral torsion is present and one side of the sacral base is found to be posterior this ligament will be under constant tension and maybe tender when palpated.

5. Iliolumbar ligament: attaches to the transverse processes of L4 and L5 and the inner border of the ilium. **Function**: limits movement of the lumbosacral junction by stabilizing the connection between the pelvis and the lower lumbar vertebrae.

Muscles and the SIJ

No muscles pass directly over the SIJ, but ligaments alone cannot maintain a stable pelvic girdle. They rely on several muscle systems to assist them: the inner core unit - (pelvic floor muscles, diaphragm, multifidi and TA) and the outer slings consisting of muscles that are anatomically and functionally related. For our purposes we'll concentrate on the posterior oblique sling: the GMax and the contralateral thoracolumbar fascia/latissimus dorsi.

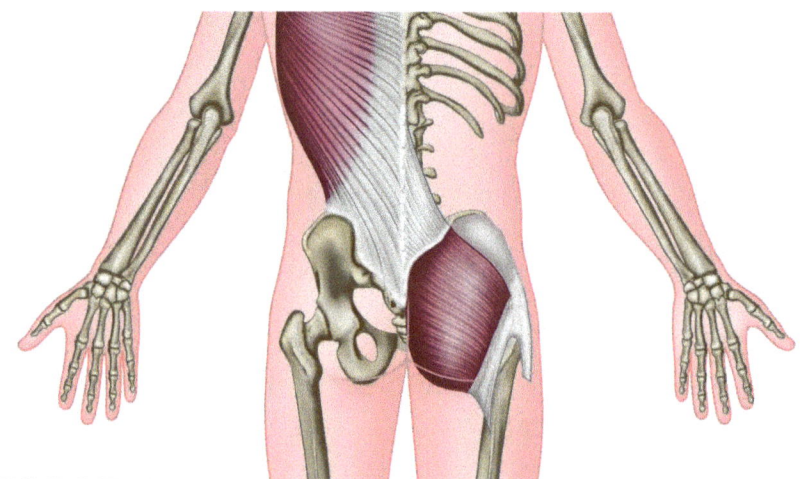

FORCE closure: Posterior sling (Gmax, contralateral thoracolumbar fascia, latissimus dorsi)

Gmax is particularly important in SIJ stabilization. It assists in self-locking and controls nutation. Some fibers merge and attach to the sacrotuberous ligament, the key ligament in SIJ stabilization, and the thoracolumbar fascial via the aponeurosis of the erector spinae.

The gluteus maximus appears to become inhibited when the SIJ is irritated or in dysfunction. Weak and/or misfiring of Gmax can have catastrophic consequences on gait – the stride length shortens and the hamstrings are overused to compensate for loss of hip extensor power and will predispose the SIJ to injury. A common reason for weakness and/or misfiring of Gmax is an overly-facilitated iliopsoas and rectus femoris.

The piriformis muscles attach to the anterior surface of the sacrum and

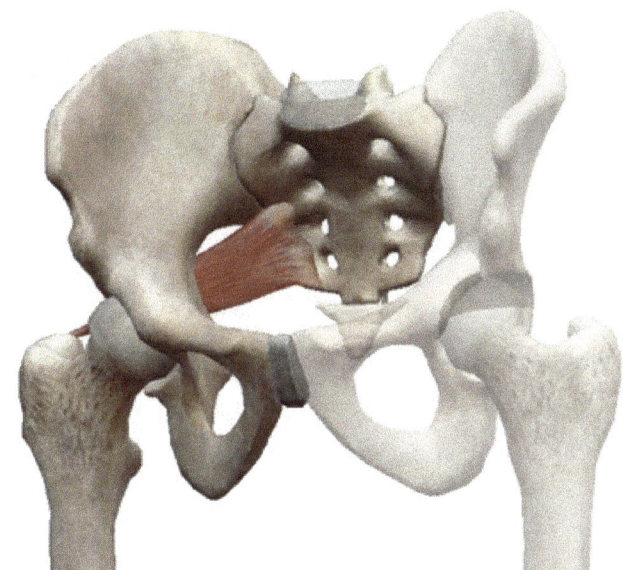

shares connective tissue across this surface. An imbalance in one piriformis is almost certainly impacting its sister. Therefore it is always important to treat both piriformis muscles when there is an issue with the sacrum.

Because the piriformis partially originates from the sacrospinous ligament, which is fascially linked to the hamstrings, trauma or overuse can create adhesive scar tissue that shortens the piriformis and drags on the sacrum. Prolonged unilateral sacral drag leads to ligament hypermobility, inflammation and sacroiliac imbalance. When the hamstrings and piriformis destabilize the SI joint, nerves (sciatic, superior and inferior gluteal) can become inflamed, causing symptoms resembling piriformis syndrome.

Piriformis can pull the sacral base posterior and inferior in a diagonal direction relative to the innominate bone and can cause wedging of sacrum against the innominate resulting in loss of mobility of SIJ.

When a client presents with a sacral torsion the deep side will have a functional shortened piriformis on that side. In this circumstance, it is again important to perform therapeutic manual techniques to both piriformis muscles and also stretch the short side. (Caution: if your client/patient is currently in piriformis syndrome, be extremely cautious when stretching. Positional release/Strain/Counterstrain are excellent conservative modalities to use before stretching.)

Assessment Tests

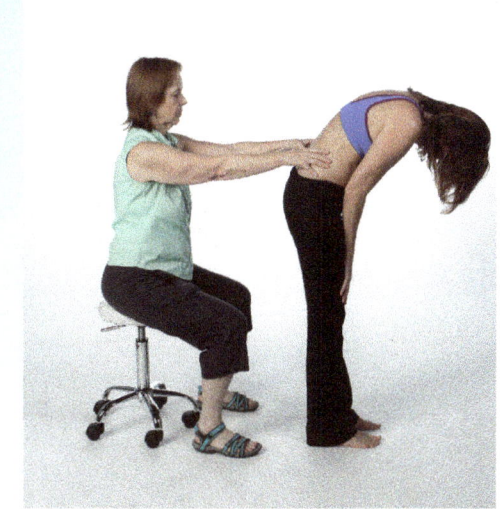

Assessment Tests

The following assessments are presented in order of increasing complexity. That is, it is common to have a high Ilium but much less common to have a sacral torsion (deep sulcus). A client with a sacral torsion will usually have a positive test for all the assessments prior to it.

For all assessments tests:

- Be at eye level with the structure being assessed
- Use dominant eye
- Extend elbows (where applicable)

1. Test for high Iliac crest

A high iliac crest will collide with the transverse process(es) of the lumbar vertebrae above it. To compensate, the vertebrae(s) will rotate away from the high ilium side and side-bend towards it. This results in a cascading effect up the spine.

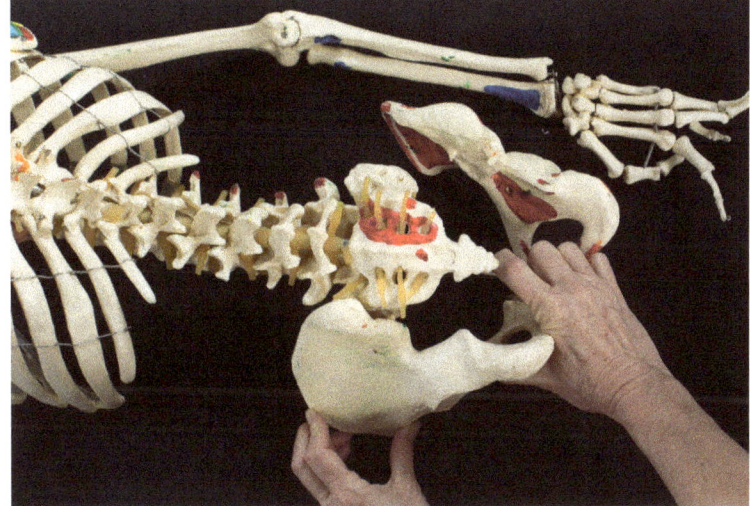

Impact of high ilium: Alters weight transfer through low back, pelvis and legs; alters force loads at the SI joint; low back pain; sciatica; increased facet joint compression; nerve compression; early arthritic changes; can reduce the opening of the intervertebral foramen leading to nerve root compression; chronic greater trochanteric bursitis.

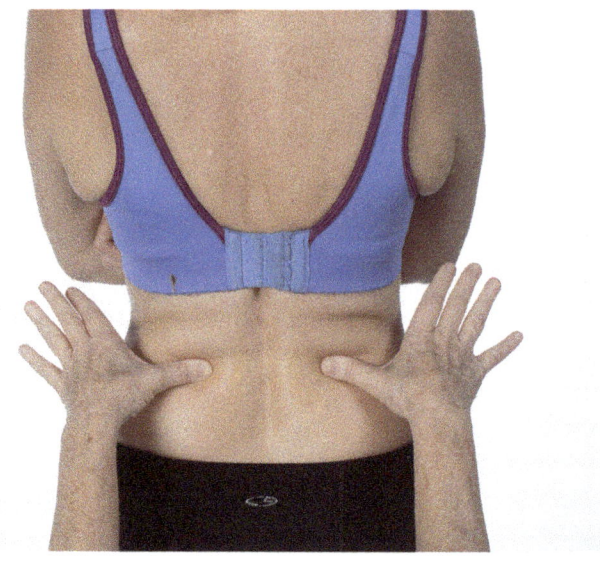
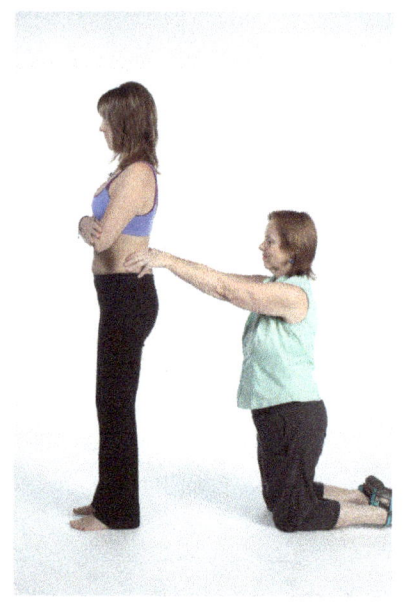

Above: Standing Test. Notice that the therapist's right thumb is slightly higher than her left thumb indicating a high right ilium.

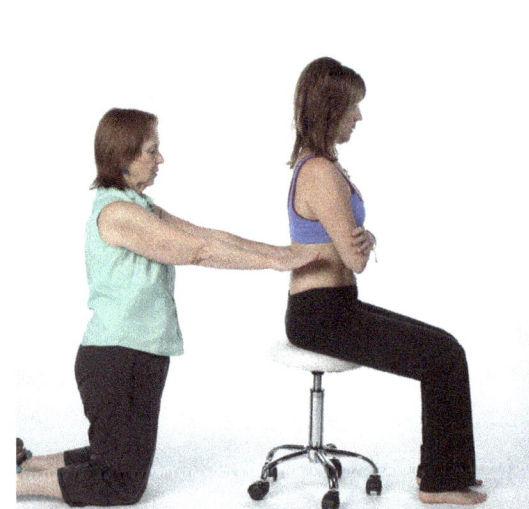
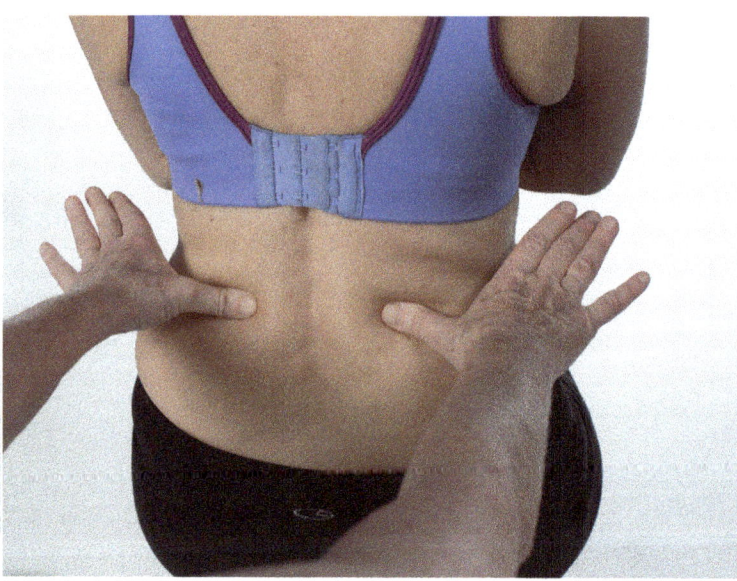

Above: Seated Test. In the seated position notice that right ilium is still slightly higher indicating that the primary muscles to address are superior to (above) the ilium — usually the quadratus lumborum.

1. Kneeling behind client, rest thumbs on either side of the spine on the iliac crest. Notice if one ilium is higher than its counterpart.

2. If one side is higher it may indicate a true or functional leg length difference.

3. If one hip is high, the test may be repeated seated. This takes the lower extremity out of the equation.

Interpretation: When a client is seated, the muscles of the lower extremities relax and cease their impact on the pelvis. Eliminating their influence on the pelvic region can provide a clearer understanding of the forces affecting the ilia.

Therefore, if the iliac crests are at different heights standing and become level seated then the primary forces influencing the deviation are below the ilium.

If the iliac crests are at different heights both standing AND seated then the primary muscles to address are superior to (above) the ilium — usually the quadratus lumborum. In other words, the QL is exerting an upward pull on that ilium.

2. Test for anterior or posterior rotation (pelvic tilt)

An innominate may rotate (around axis X) to be either anterior or posterior.

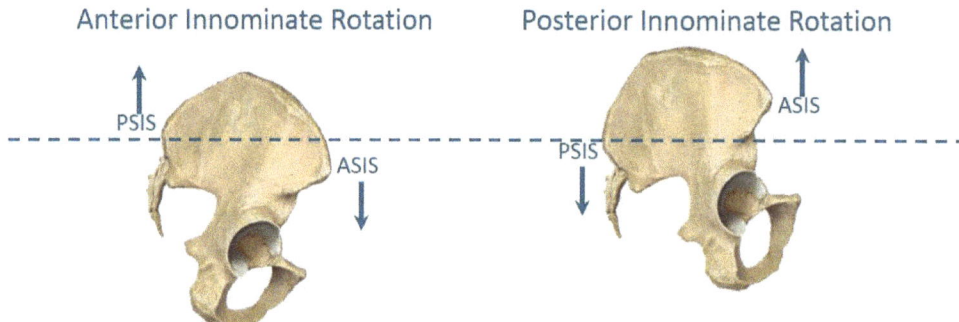

In fact, an anterior innominate (especially the right) is the most common misalignment in the pelvis. A high iliac crest will almost always be present as well.

Impact of anterior rotation: increased lumbar lordosis; displacement of 5th lumbar vertebrae; strain on the SIJ often times leading to an upslip; functional leg length difference may result; chronic greater trochanteric bursitis.

We'll use the relationship of two bony landmarks, the anterior superior iliac spine (ASIS) and the posterior superior iliac spine (PSIS). As a general rule, the ASIS varies from directly anterior of the PSIS to 1/2 inch inferior of the PSIS. Deviations within this range are considered normal. If the ASIS is more than 1/2 inch inferior to the PSIS the client has an excessive anterior rotation. If the ASIS is superior to the PSIS the client has a posterior rotation of the pelvis.

1. Client is standing. Kneel at the side of the client. Place one finger on the center of her PSIS. Find the PSIS by placing your thumbs on the posterior medial section of the ilium. Lower your thumbs about 1/2 inch. Feel for the dimples that most people have. Just beneath these dimples, feel for a small bony protuberance. This is the PSIS. It takes a bit of practice — if you've never done it before, be bold and ask your friends and family to participate in a palpation exercise.

2. Find the ASIS by placing your finger on the anterior medial portion of the iliac crest. The ASIS will be just inferior to your fingers. You may ask your client to lean forward (trunk flexion) to help find the ASIS. Hook your finger under her ASIS.

3. Lean back and extend your elbows.

4. Test the other side.

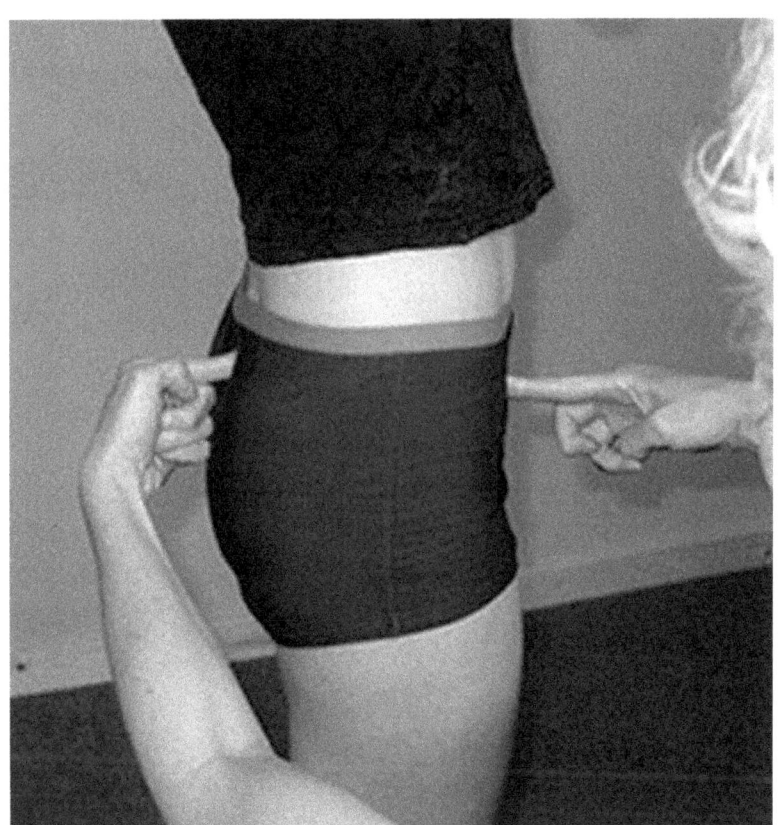

3. Sacroiliac Joint — Test for upslipped innominate

Sacroiliac upslips (upward shearing force of ilium on sacrum) are more affected by gravity than any other sacral distortion with a limited chance of self-correction. Clients often report symptoms to be more painful than expected from the injury they experienced. Prolonged altered loading can interfere with both force and form closure to the point that an act as innocent as slamming on the car brakes can jostle the joint enough to cause it to misalign and force closure cannot take place. The SIJ can undergo fibrous fusion in later life. Movement of SIJ decreases with age.

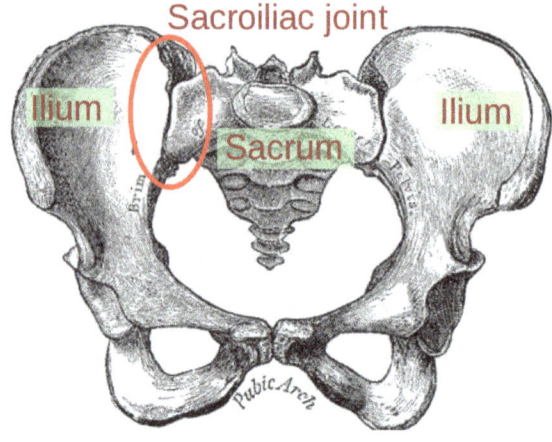

Impact of upslip: Muscle spasms; ligament laxity; altered weight transfer; difficulty walking; neural compression; sciatica; pain when rising from sitting.

If a client tests positive for both high ilium and anterior rotation, there is a good chance that there will also be an upslip.

1. Client is standing. Locate the PSIS. Find the PSIS by placing your thumbs on the superior medial section of the posterior pelvis. Lower your thumbs about 1/2 inch, then move them about a 1/2 inch laterally. Feel for the dimples that most people have. Just beneath these dimples, feel for a small bony protuberance. This is the PSIS. Move the thumbs just inferior so you are on the lower edge of the PSIS.

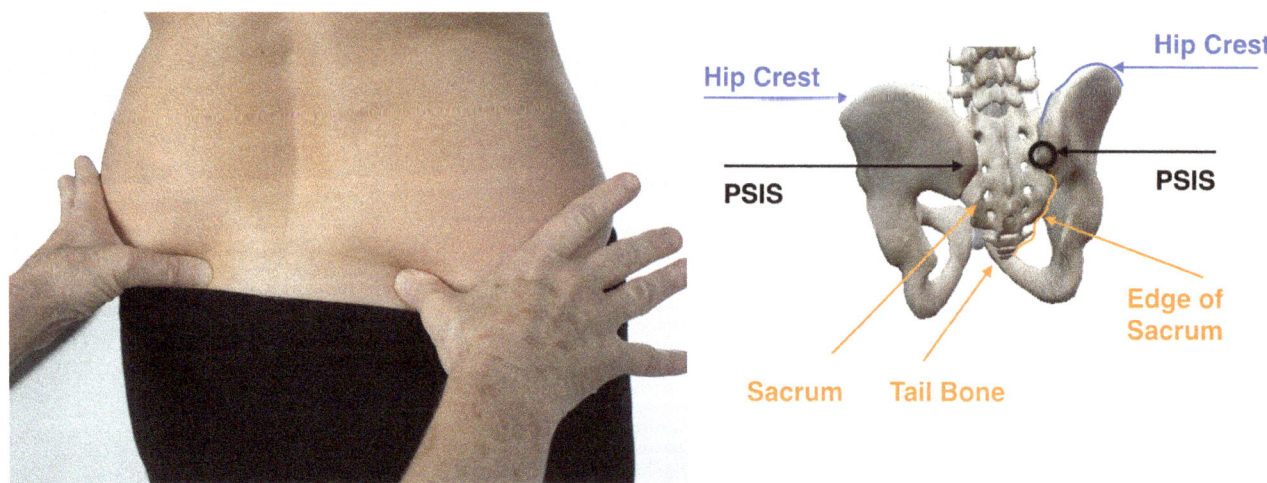

2. Cue the client to perform a slow spinal flexion: Tuck chin to chest and slowly roll down towards the floor. This spinal flexion should take about five seconds. There should be no bend in the knees because you'll get a false reading. Therapist maintains contact on PSIS.

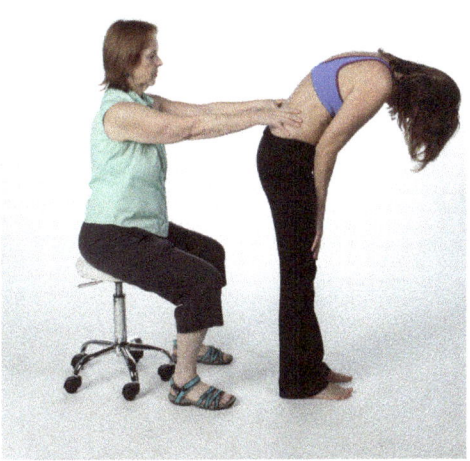

3. The practitioner observes, especially near the end of the spinal flexion, whether one thumb (and PSIS) starts to move upwards before the other. The dysfunctional side is that on which the thumb moves first during flexion.

Interpretation: If one thumb moves superiorly during flexion it indicates that the ilium is fixed to the sacrum on that side.

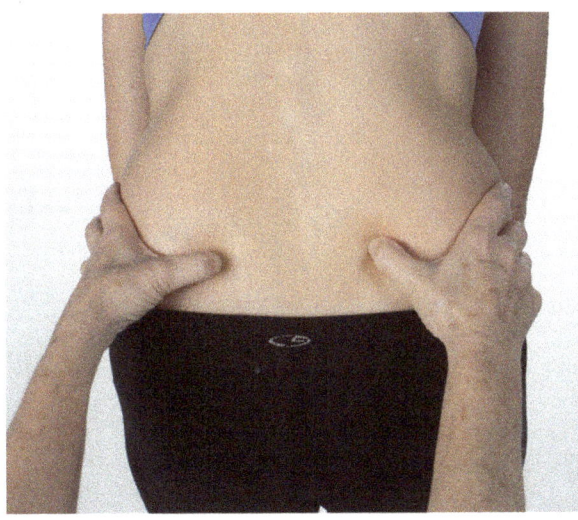

Left: Notice the therapist's right thumb is higher on right indicating a positive upslip test on right ilium.

When a positive flexion test is found in standing we know the ilium and sacrum are "stuck" on that side but we don't know why. It could be a true leg length difference or a rotated ilium or a sacral torsion.

4. Test for leg length difference (medial malleoli)

This test is done to gather additional information and is not related to a particular correction. It lets us know if there is a disturbance in the pelvis by comparing leg length supine and seated.

Many people will test or appear to have a leg length difference. However for ninety percent of the population it is functional rather than true leg length difference. A misalignment in the pelvis causes the leg to appear shorter when it really isn't. Once the pelvic issue is resolved, the legs should match in length.

Tests for true leg length difference can be technical, expensive and complex. This technique is simple, free and highly accurate. It is most useful for measuring larger differences of ¼ inch or more.

1. The client is supine. Have the client do a bridge to bring the pelvis into neutral. The therapist places her thumbs on the inner ankle bones (medial malleoli). Compare the thumbs noting if they are level.

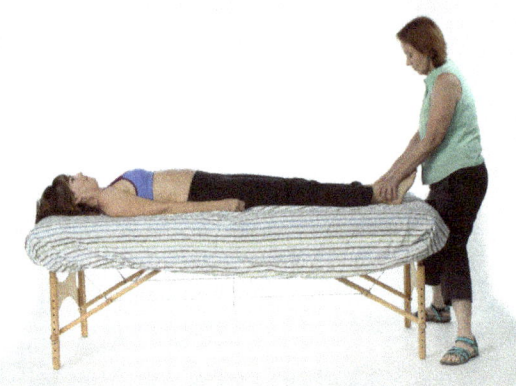

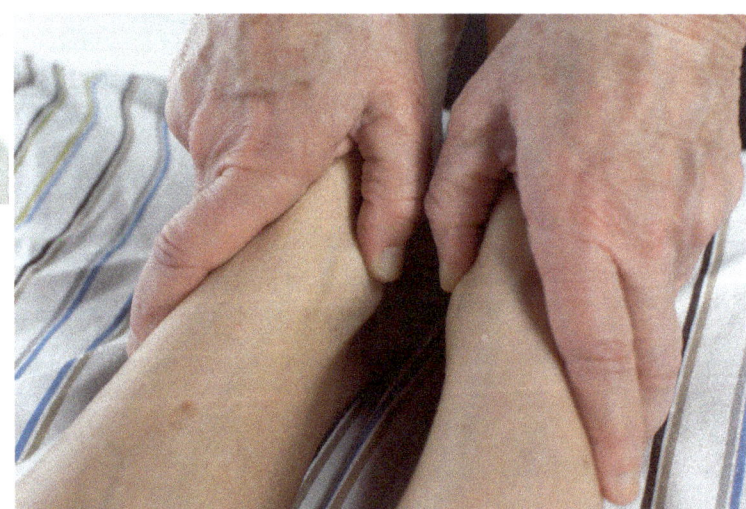

Above: Note thumbs are level in supine postion.

2. Cue the client sit up on the table, legs still extended, and recheck the malleoli. Keep your thumbs on the malleoli throughout the test. As the client sits up, observe whether one ankle draws up as opposed to the opposite lengthening down.

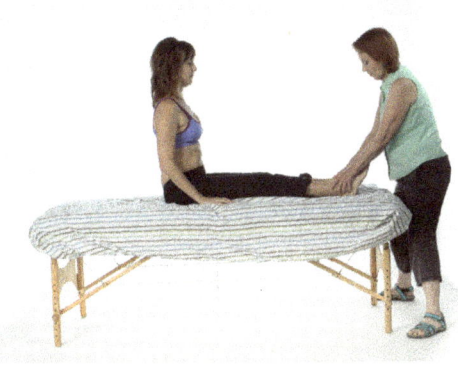

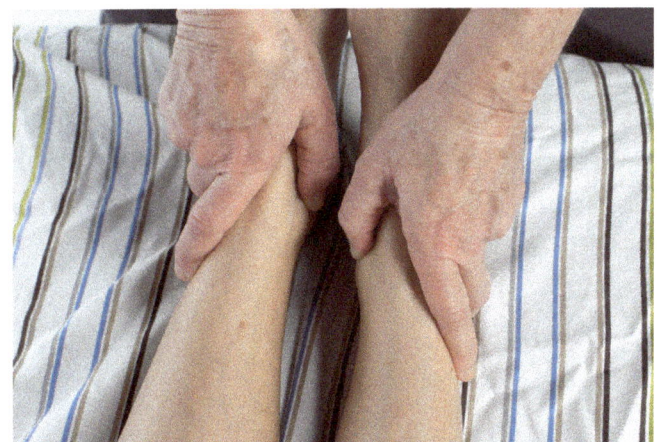

Above: Note that client's right malleolus is higher than left in seated position indicating root cause is coming from pelvis.

Interpretation*: If the medial malleoli changed relative to each other between these two checks, we know that the root cause of the apparent leg length difference is coming from the pelvis. It could be an anteriorly rotated (tilted) inominate, upslip or sacral torsion. A leg length difference that is maintained both seated and supine would indicate the difference originates in the lower extremity and is a true leg length difference. Ask clients if they had an injury to the knees, legs, ankles and usually they have had a major injury.
*Differences of 1/8 or less not significant for such a basic test

This is a great test to recheck after your session to notice the seemingly miraculous correction of a short leg!

5. Pubic Symphysis Test

Impact of misalignment of pubic symphysis: Symptoms might include radiating pain into the back, abdomen, groin, perineum or legs; tenderness at the pubic symphsis or SI joints; loss of strength during aDduction of the thighs or a "waddling" walk due to the aDduction weakness.

The pubic symphysis is a cartilaginous joint with a fibrous disc reinforced by a series of ligaments. During pregnancy the gap widens 2-3 mm. In men the gap is smaller and narrower.

In severe cases a medical condition called pubic symphysis dysfunction can occur – an MRI or Xray might be used to diagnose. For our purposes we will use either a palpation or a strength test of the aDductors to determine if a pubic bone distortion may be present.

1. Client is supine (no bolster under knees). Have the client do a bridge to bring the pelvis into neutral. Therapist stands at the head or side of the table places thumbs just above client's pubic symphysis. Compare the thumbs noting if they are level.

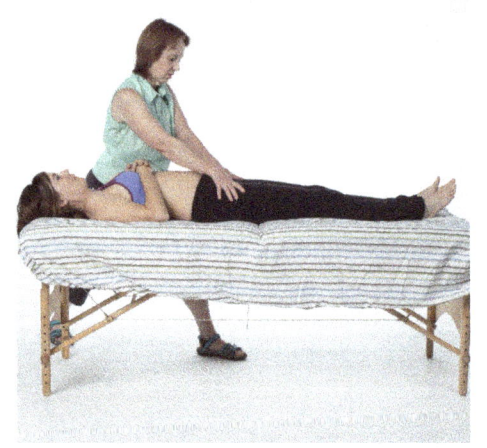
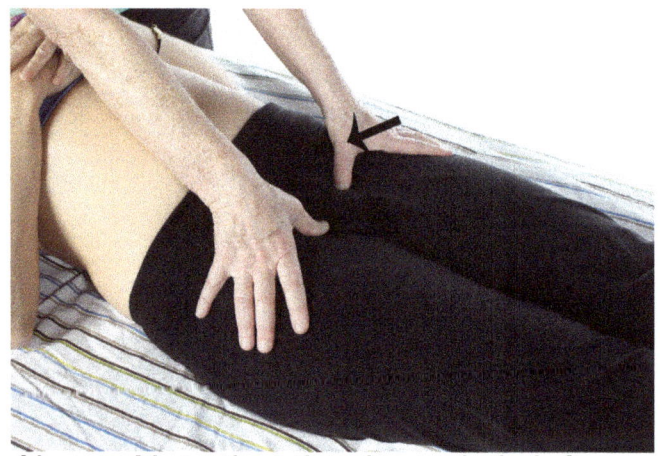

Above: Note that the therapist's left thumb is higher than right indicating a misalignment in the pubic symphysis.

Interpretation: If one thumb is higher (superior) this may indicate a misalignment of the pubic symphysis.

It may be more comfortable for the client to have knees bent and feet on the table. However, we find it easier to "get a reading" with legs out straight.

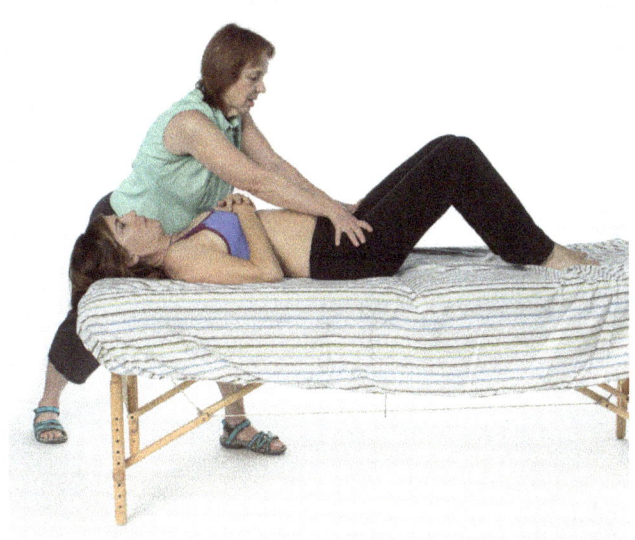

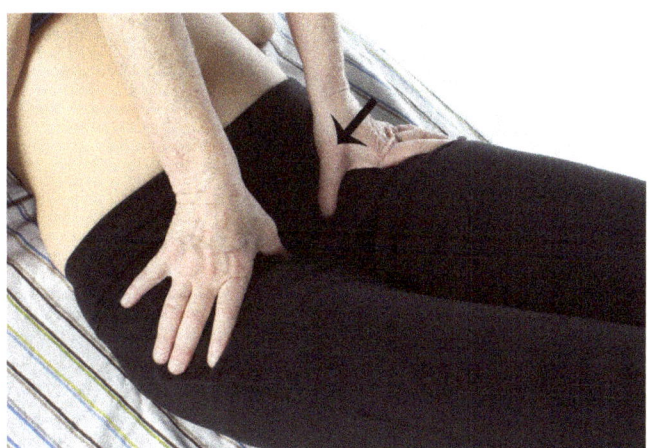

Above: Note that the therapist's left thumb is higher than right indicating a misalignment is the pubic symphysis.

6. Test for Sacral Torsion

Impact of sacral torsion: Unlevel sacral base; rotoscoliosis or corkscrewing of structures all the way to O-A joint; piriformis spasm (deep sulcus is usually on side of tight piriformis); sciatica; ligament laxity; inflammation.

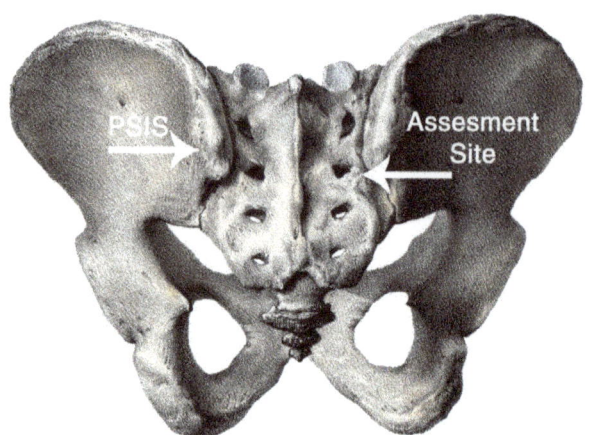

This test may be done prone or seated. If the client is prone, feet are off the table and forehead rests on hands. This position puts the spine in a neutral posture. The sacral sulcus can be a bit tricky to find. Sometimes it helps to have the client do a "mini" cobra (spine hyperextension).

Palpating for sacral torsion:
1. Begin by finding both right and left PSIS.

2. From the PSIS move slightly medial so that you are now on the sacrum and off the ilia. Feel for a hollow area (sometimes referred to as the sacral sulcus).

3. Place an *index* finger directly over the site and press straight into the body. Press the fingers simultaneously so that tautness of superficial tissue does not impact your assessment. Notice if either finger sinks in deeper than the other.

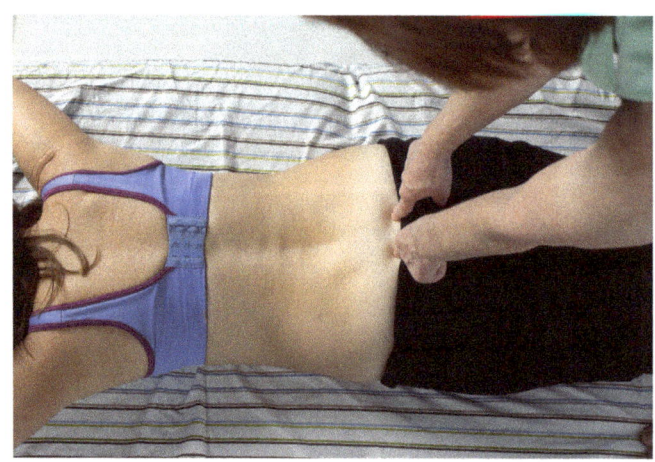

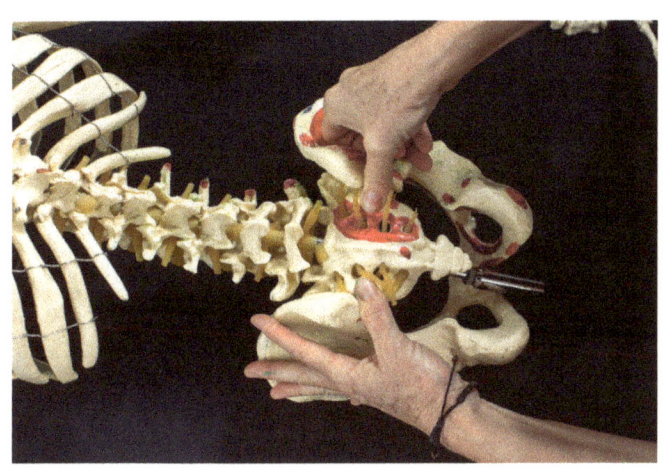
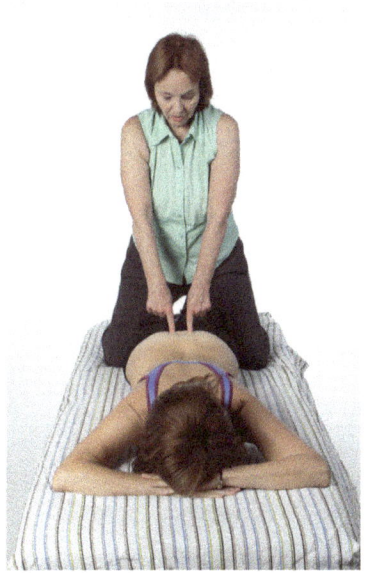

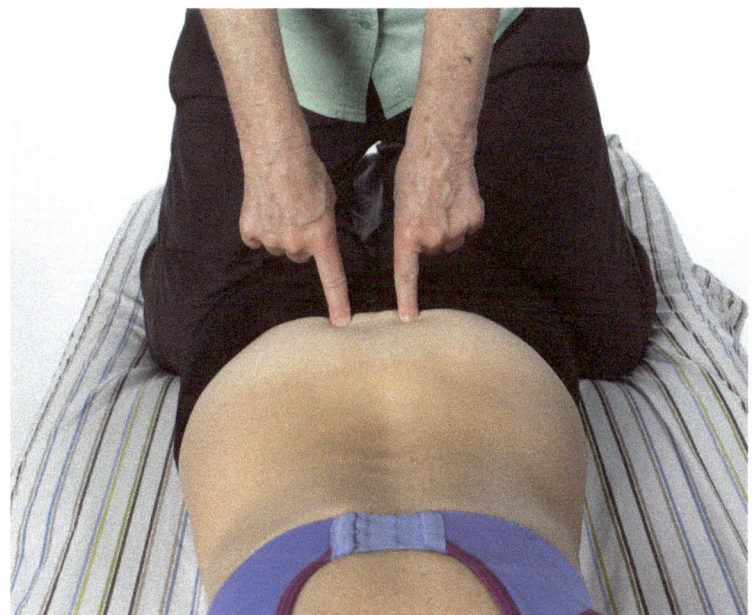

Above: Notice that the therapist's right index finger is deeper than her left indicating a deep right or anteriorly rotated right sulcus.

Interpretation: This is termed a "deep sulcus" or an anteriorly rotated side of the sacrum. The opposite side is posteriorly rotated and the sacral base is unlevel. If there is a sacral torsion the client will have most of the other misalignments.

Muscle Energy Techniques

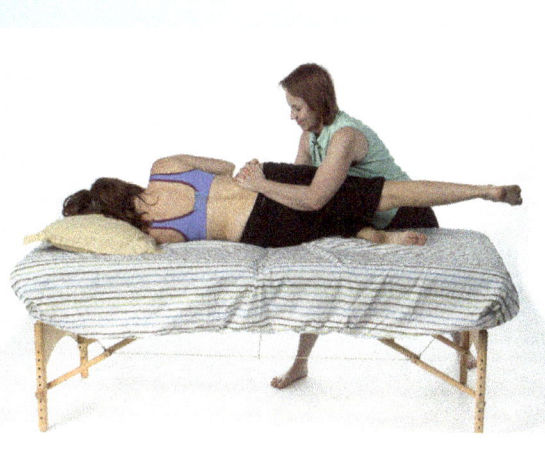

Muscle Energy Techniques

Bone is the slave of the muscle

MET methods all employ variations on a basic theme: Using the patient's own muscular effort usually while the therapist resists the effort. The practitioner's force exactly matches the effort of the client allowing no movement to occur. In other words, an isometric contraction.

This produces a contraction resulting in reciprocal inhibition of the antagonist and post-isometric relaxation of the agonist (muscle(s) that are concentrically contracted, locked short and overly-facilitated.) This neurological response (via the Golgi tendon organs and muscle spindles) "takes it to the brain". A global response is produced rather than a peripheral response.

MET may be employed to relax tight, tense muscles (antagonist/agonist contract strategies in stretching) spasms (antagonist contract), and also helps in reducing the fibrotic restrictions in chronic soft tissue problems. However, we will be using it in a specific way involving bony position and joints. We combine these corrections with soft tissue work to enhance the client's ability to hold the corrections when she returns to weight-bearing and activities of daily living.

No matter how good a manual therapist someone is, she will have limited results on soft tissue until skeletal misalignments are addressed. Unlike chiropractic thrust techniques, MET uses the body's muscles to pull the bones back into alignment. These corrections combined with soft tissue work allow the client to return to weight bearing and activities of daily living.

BENEFITS OF MET

1. Maximum precision and minimum force
2. Relaxes muscles
3. Mobilizes restricted joints
4. Strengthens inhibited muscles
5. Reduces local edema
6. Stretches muscles and fascia
7. Resets muscle spindles and golgi tendon organs

End Range of Movement

The End of Range (EOR) of movement is the physiological barrier of a joint. It is the stopping point past which a joint cannot be passively moved without applying force. The end of the movement could be from muscles bumping into each other (as in flexing the knee), soft tissue reaching its end of stretch (dorsiflexion of the ankle), bone meeting bone (elbow extension) or capsular or ligamentous stretching (internal rotation of the femur for example).

There are also abnormal or pathological reasons for EOR such as inflammation or arthritis. In any case, the recipient should never feel pain in the joint from the positioning of EOR. MET may be contraindicated for people with arthritis or hyper-mobility issues.

To treat joint restrictions with MET, follow these simple guidelines:

1. Instruct the client to breathe throughout the technique.

2. Slowly position the joint at EOR (first physiological barrier).

3. Instruct the client to statically contract the muscles towards their freedom of motion (away from EOR) as the practitioner resists any movement of the joint (agonist contract).

4. The client uses about 20% of strength. A good way to kinesthetically cue the client is "Push into my hand and match my pressure." The client holds this isometric contraction for about 5-10 seconds.

5. Cue the client to relax (post-isometirc relaxation). The practitioner re-engages the joint at its new EOR and holds the correction for 15 seconds.

6. Repeat steps 3-5 until free movement is achieved or no further gain is apparent. Usually 3 repetitions.

Corrections (In this order)

In order to maximize the body's ability to hold the corrections, they are done in this order. The larger more powerful muscles are released and the major bone misalignments are addressed first. This allows the pelvis and surrounding tissues to return to a more neutral position.

Only perform those corrections that had a positive test.

Practitioner may retest after each correction or, if multiple corrections are performed, may retest at the end.

1A. High Iliac Crest Correction

1. Client lies on her side with HIGH iliac crest down, knees bent.

2. Therapist slides the knees toward the chest until the L5 spinal process begins to move.

3. Gently move lower legs toward ceiling until end of range is felt. Do a posterior traction of top hip if needed.

4. Do three rounds of MET with client pressing lower legs towards the table. After each round, therapist gently moves feet toward ceiling to next EOR.

Cuing client as to which muscles should fire can be helpful. Therapist may tap on QL to give client a proprioceptive cue.

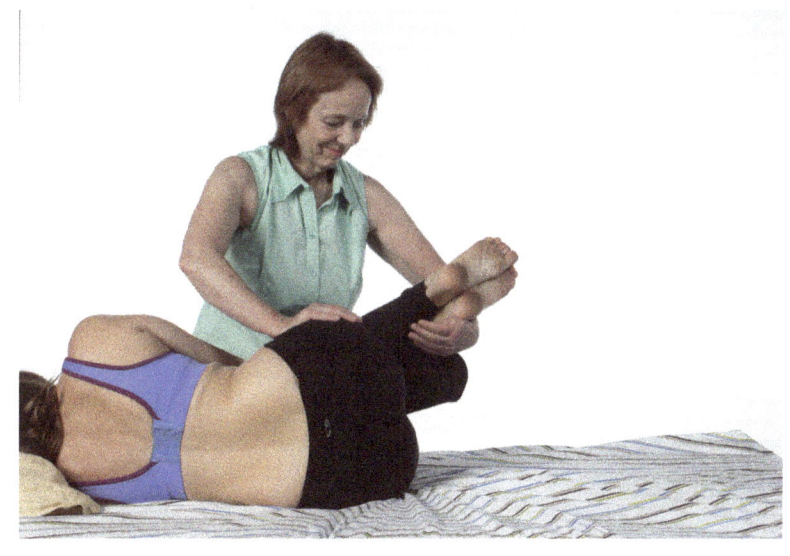

1B. Alternative method

In some cases, the above method causes pain in the hip, groin or knee. If so, the following alternative can be used.

1. Client in side lying position with affected side up.

2. Therapist grasps ilium with hands interlocked and forearms squeezing thigh.

3. Therapist gently pulls the ilium toward the foot of the table to EOR.

4. The client lifts upper leg toward the ceiling.

3. Repeat three (or more) rounds of MET moving to new EOR after each round.

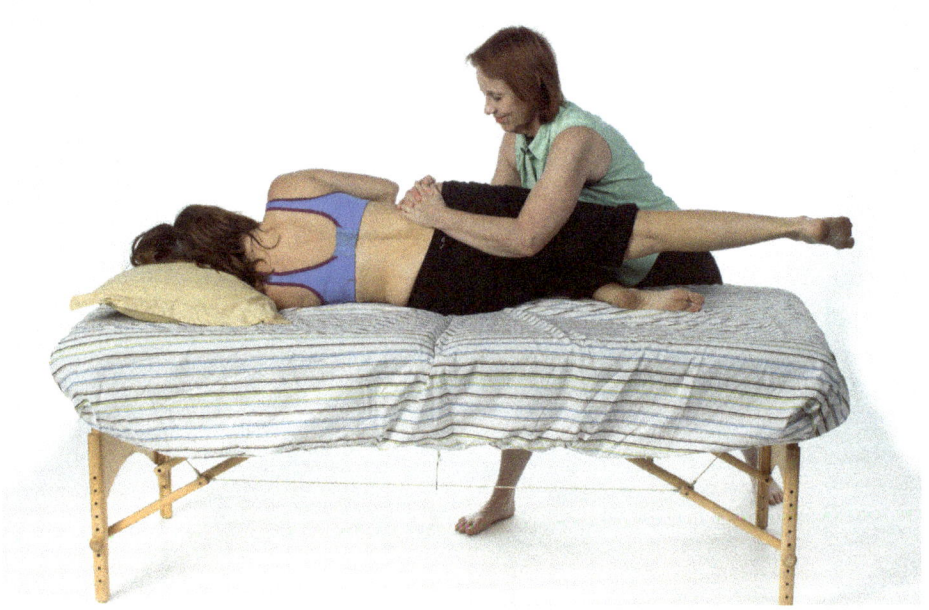

2 A. Anterior Pelvic Rotation Correction

1. Client is supine. Therapist flexes affected thigh to ninety degrees.

2. Traction the femur of the affected leg up towards the ceiling then angle the thigh to the outside (externally rotate). Return thigh to neutral and increase the degree of thigh flexion. This maneuver creates space in the thigh joint which helps eliminate the impingement of structures within the joint. Therapist bends affected-side knee into client's chest to EOR.

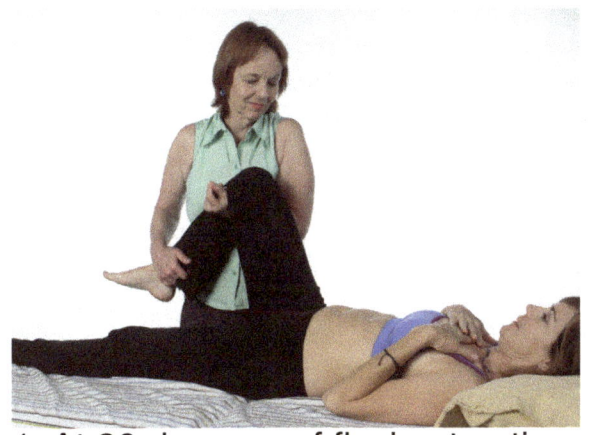

1. At 90 degrees of flexion traction thigh towards ceiling.

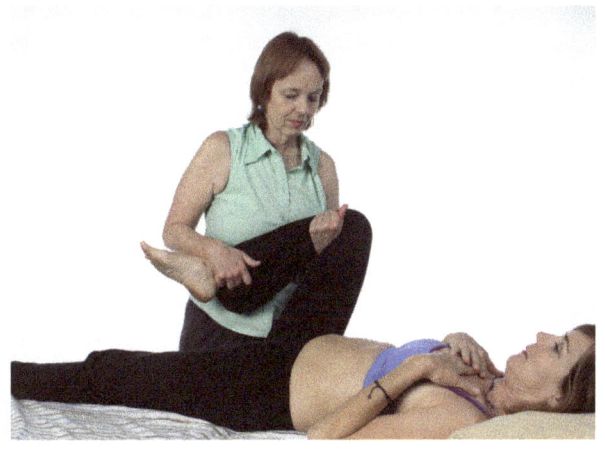

2. Externally rotate the thigh.

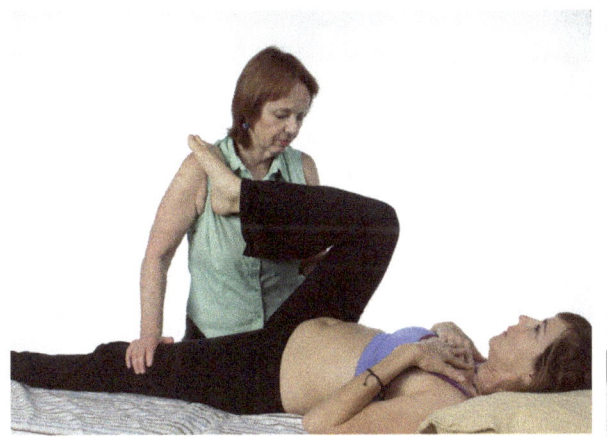

3. Return thigh to neutral and increase the degree of thigh flexion. Place hand on opposite thigh to stabilize.

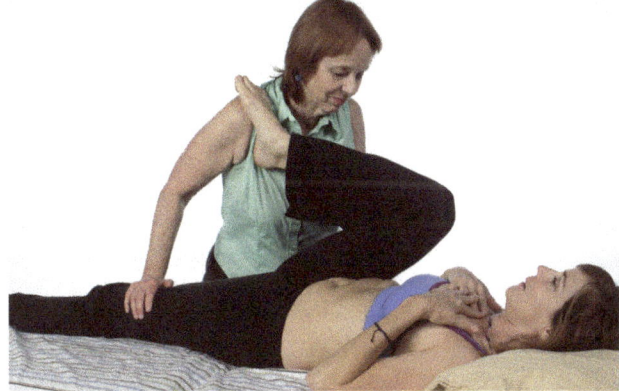

4. Client's foot is placed on therapist's shoulder and client is instructed to push foot into therapist. Gluteus maximus and hamstrings engage thus creating forced closure of SIJ.

5. MET is repeated moving to new EOR after each repetition.

2 B. Anterior Pelvic Rotation Correction Variation

This variation is great for folks who cannot flex their thighs above 90 degrees.

1. Client is supine. Client places feet flat on table so that thighs and knees are in a comfortable amount of flexion.

2. Therapist places hands over the client's ASIS on the affected side.

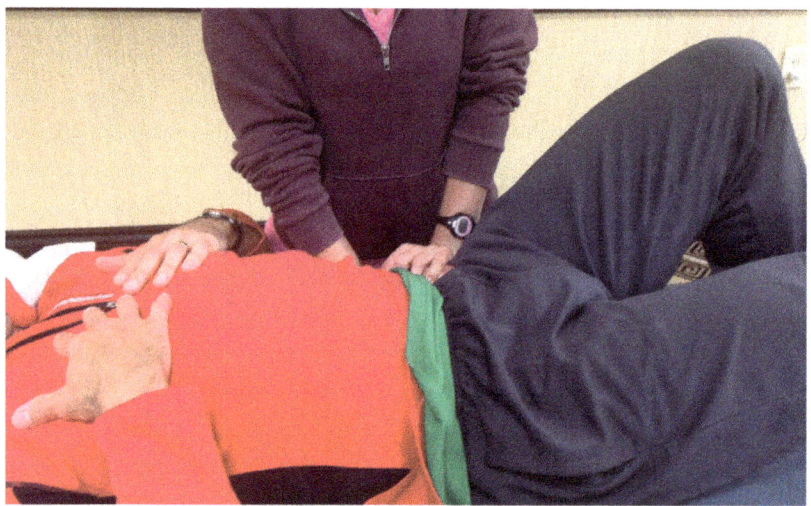

3. Client performs an anterior pelvic tilt while the therapists resists the movement. (Photo above)

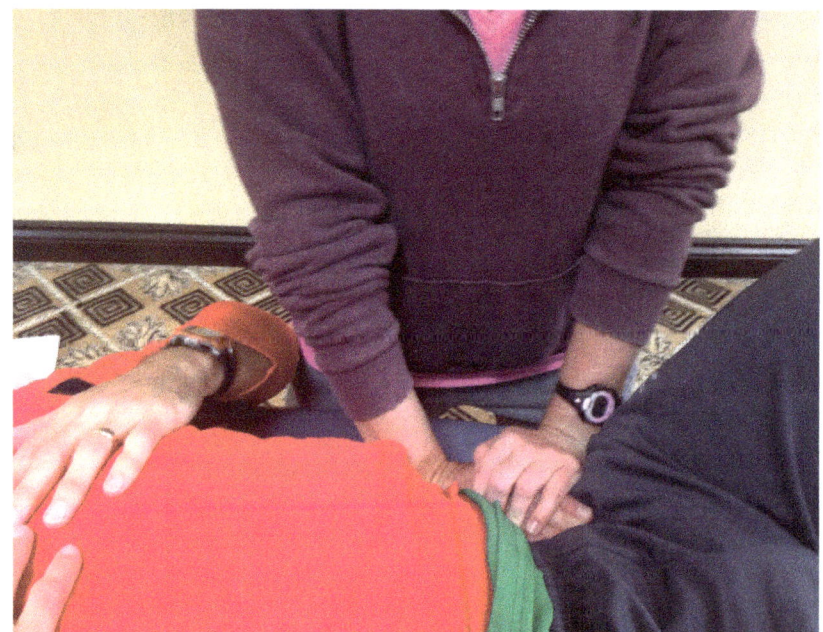

4. Therapist gently pushes anteriorly rotated side into a posterior tilt to EOR. Client is passive. (Photo above)

3. Sacroiliac Upslip Corrrection

1. Client lies supine with the affected side knee bent and foot on table.

2. Therapist slides inside arm under the client's knee and places outside hand on thigh to securely arm-lock the thigh. Therapist lifts foot of affected side about an inch off the table and internally rotates thigh until EOR to lock the SIJ.

3. Simultaneously, the client draws affected hip towards head (hip-hike) and therapist tractions leg. After a few seconds ask client to cough several times. Traction combined with forced exhalations allows the ilium to drop down into the groove.

4. Repeat MET three times, lengthening and internally rotating to next EOR after each round. The EOR change is subtle with this correction.

Note: If the above is not successful, ensure that step 2 is executed accurately and the leg is internally rotated to the point that the SIJ is locked.

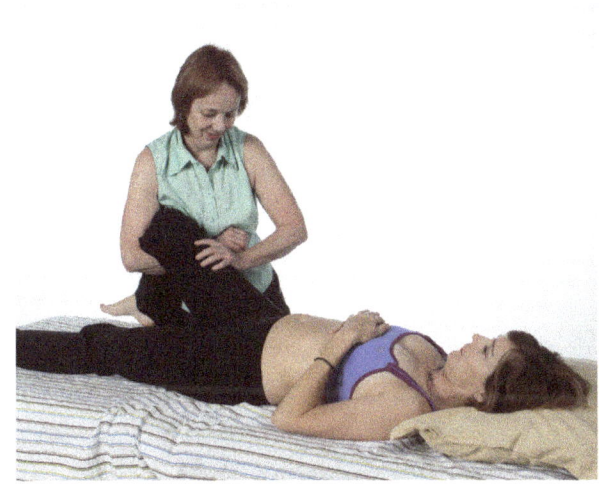

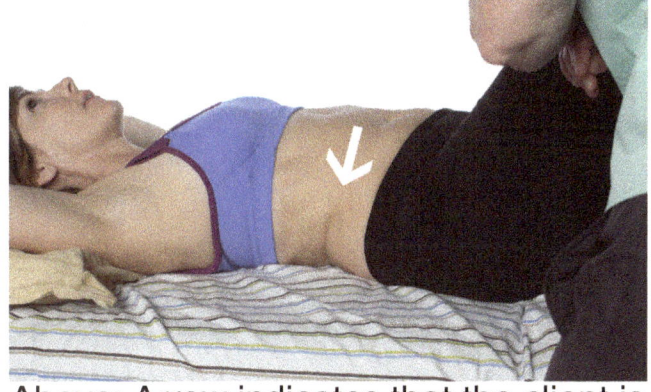

Above: Arrow indicates that the client is hiking her right ilium.

Note: this correction can also be done with the client in a side-lying position. Follow the directions for the supine correction.

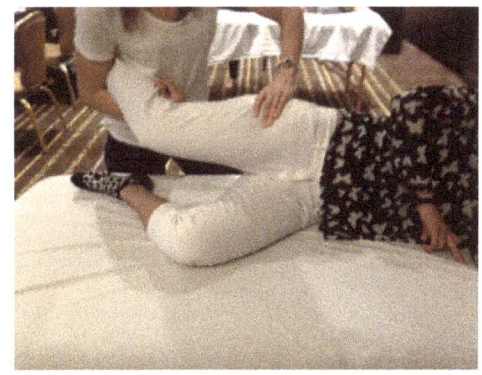

4. Pubic Symphysis Correction

1. Client is supine with knees bent and feet near buttocks. Client does slight posterior tilt of pelvis.

2. The therapist places hands on interior aspect of knees in a cross-hand position. Or entire forearm with hand on one inner knee and elbow on the opposite inner knee.

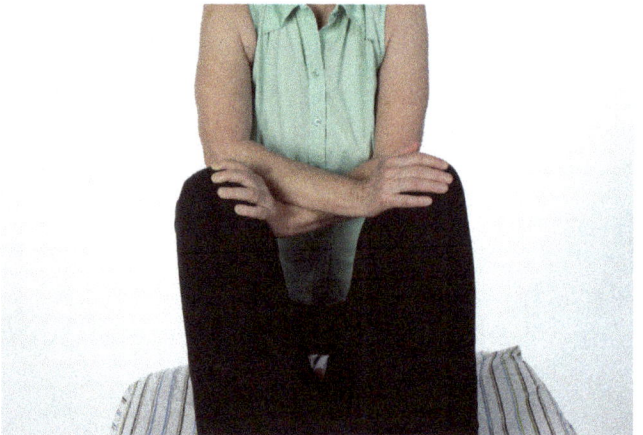

3. The client squeezes the knees towards each other (resisted adduction). Unlike most MET, full strength is used.

Alternative method

If the above does not resolve the misalignment, the following "Shotgun" technique may work.

1. Client is supine with legs flat on table and aBducted.

2. The therapist places hands on inner aspect of thighs just above knees.

3. Client squeezes quickly (one second) and with full strength. *Unlike most MET, full strength is used.*

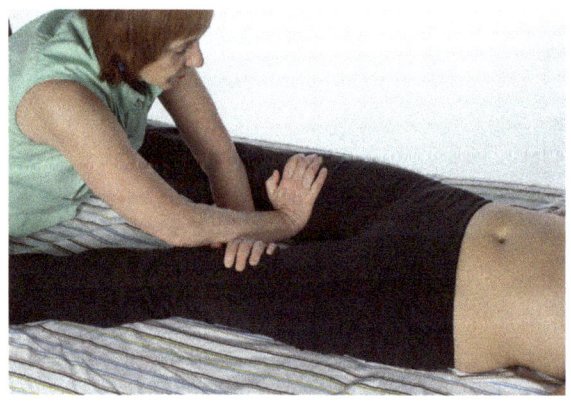

5. Sacral Torsion Correction

1. Client is lying on the deep sulcus side. Knees are bent.

2. Rotate the upper torso posteriorly as far is it will go without moving the hips. The spine will revolve all the way down to L5 and may require the upper arm to be behind back.

3. With one hand on the client's sacrum, slide the knees toward the head until the sacrum moves. Then straighten the bottom leg.

4. Lift the ankle and calf of the top leg toward the ceiling until EOR. Keep the top thigh level with the table

5. Client attempts to push ankle toward table while therapist adds resistance. Repeat three rounds of MET. Client uses only 10% of strength as opposed to the 20% usually used. Therapist draws top foot towards the ceiling to new EOR after each repetition.

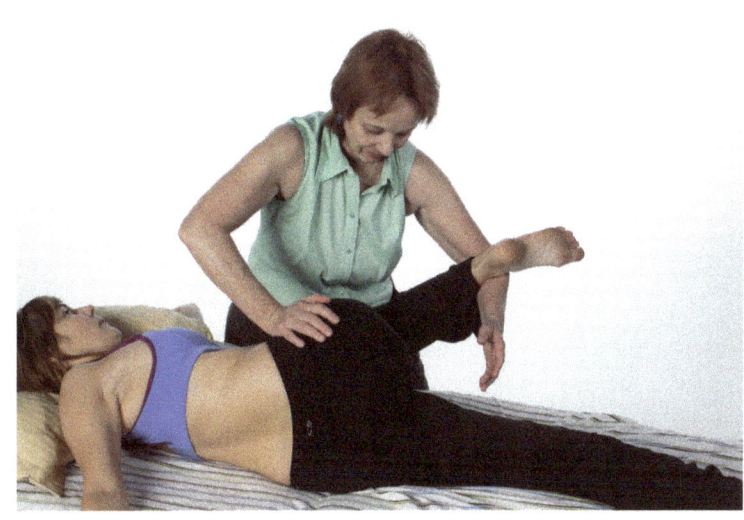

Note: If the correction does not work ensure the upper body is fully rotated to L5 and thighs are flexed until sacrum moves.

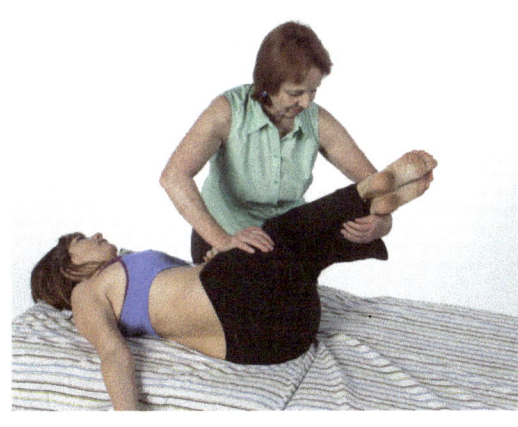

If the above correction is still not successful, repeat with both legs bent and lift both ankles as shown in photo left.

Muscle Swimming Deep Tissue Techniques

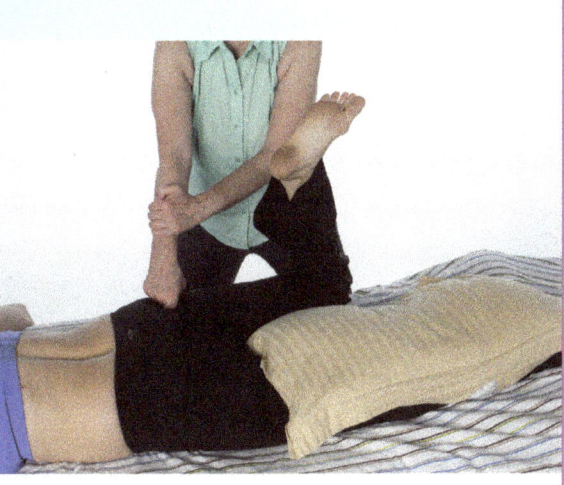

Principles of Muscle Swimming

> It's all about the principles! "As to methods there may be a million and then some, but principles are few. The man who grasps principles can successfully select his own methods. The man who tries methods, ignoring principles is sure to have trouble."
> (Ralph Waldo Emerson)

As manual therapists we all face the question, "How can I best facilitate tissue release and allow the muscle to return to its happy, healthy resting state while maintaining my own ecology of movement?" I stumbled across an answer to that dilemma many years ago and have been refining my approach ever since in both my private practice and seminars. Simply put, Muscle Swimming uses physiology to facilitate release of myofascial structures allowing the therapist to work smarter and the client to have co-ownership of the session. The following are the core components of Muscle Swimming:

1. Warm the tissue with Swedish strokes before deep tissue work.

2. **Pin and Rock:** our first encounter with a stressed myofascial unit should be gentle and non-threatening. Passively shorten the muscle, gently pin it with multiple fingers for a broad, dispersed pressure and add a slow rhythmic rocking of the joint. Rocking stimulates a parasympathetic response. After all, we are rocked for nine months. In fact, the first nerves to myelinate in the human fetus are the vestibular nerves which sense movement. Our first consciousness is that we are a moving beings. Be patient – wait for the tissue to soften and yield before moving to the Pin and Move protocol. Come back to this Pin and Rock maneuver whenever you sense guarding in your client.

3. **Pin and Move:** when you meet an area of dense fascia, trigger points, tender points or just plain snarly tissue, integrate active movement. Active movement "takes it to the brain", involving the central nervous system, creating longer lasting results. Fascial layers and actin and myosin myofibrils glide across each other as the muscle goes through its shortened, neutral and stretched states.

    A. Place the muscle in a shortened state.

    B. Pin the area at first barrier. If it's a trigger point or tender point, use one finger, or appropriate tool for specificity and work it from an oblique angle of 45 degrees.

    C. Have your client do a movement. Start with the main

action the muscle performs, i.e. flexion, abduction, extension etc. Movement should be done at a slow to medium tempo.

        D. Client repeats the movement 4-5 times.

        E. Ask your client if the area or point is better, worse or the same. If your client says that the area is better, your nest question is, "how much better?" If your client reports at least a 50% change for the better, then move to another area and repeat the above steps.

        F. If your client reports no change you have three options:

            1. Add resistance to the current movement pattern. This loads the muscle and recruits more fibers, allowing you to swim through the tissue. 10 - 20% of resistance is usually all that is needed. For example, your client is performing thigh flexions while you pin a stubborn trigger point in the iliopsoas. To add resistance, simply place your downhill hand on the thigh, add 10 - 20% of resistance and ask your client to continue the thigh flexions.

2. Try another movement pattern. Adding resistance to the new pattern is always an option.

3. Ask your client for input. She may feel an itch to move the joint in a certain way.

        G. If your client reports that the point or area is worse that is not necessarily a negative outcome. It's possible that through the portal of Active Movement, you've swum to a trigger point or congested area at a deeper layer of tissue.
The same three options apply to this situation as well:

            1. Add resistance to the current movement pattern.

            2. Try another movement pattern. Adding resistance to the new pattern is always an option.

            3. Ask your client for input. She may feel an itch to move the joint in a certain way.

4. Work the muscle(s) from as many different positions as possible — supine, side-lying, prone, and even weight-bearing. Perhaps your client is a golfer suffering from low back pain and the quadratus lumborum is the main culprit. Have him go through a golf swing while you work the tissue. Think outside the

box and get the client moving!

5. When you find an exquisitely tender spot or trigger point, work to release the tissue around it before concentrating on the tender point.

6. Give your client a break! Working on these muscles, especially the iliopsoas, can be quite stressful. Incorporate what I call the "sweet stuff" during your deep tissue work, i.e., energy work, a short foot massage, some relaxing effleurage, etc.

7. Breath connects us all! Breathe deeply while working and encourage your client to do the same.

8. Combine working two muscles at the same time. Since all muscles work interdependently this is an especially effective release technique.

9. Practice patience, non-judgment, curiosity, and compassion.

10. If it hurts you, don't do it! Adapt the technique to suit your body.

Principles of Muscle Swimming

RECAP

- Warm the Tissue
- Always begin with the muscle in a shortened state
- Release the muscle in all its states – short, neutral, stretched
- Release the muscle in different positions when possible: supine,
- side-lying, prone
- Pin & Rock - client is passive
- Pin & Move - client performs active movements. This is a trial and error process. Be flexible and creative!

Benefits of Pin and Move

- Active movement takes it to the brain!
- Client experiences novel sensory information and increased proprioception
- Client becomes more somatically aware.

Muscle Swimming techniques for gluteal group and external rotators of the hip

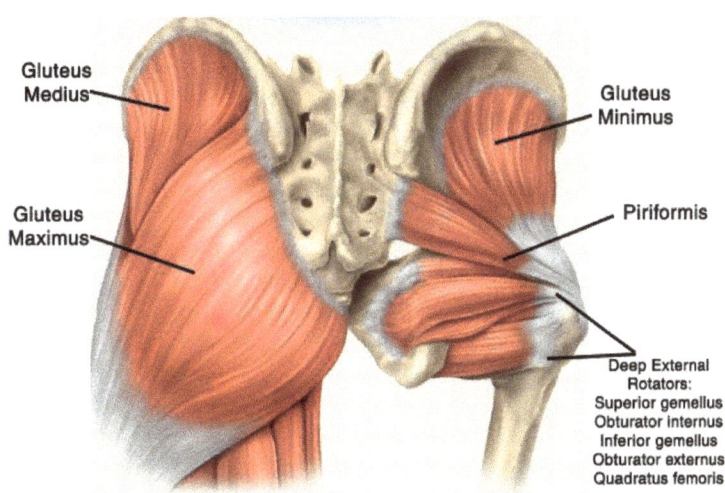

Attachments:
Gluteus maximus: lateral sacrum, thoracolumbar fascia, aponeurosis of erector spinea, iliac crest, sacroiliac and sacrotuberous ligaments and coccygeal vertebrae; inserts into gluteal tuberosity
Gluteus medius: outer surface of iliumand gluteal aponeurosis; inserts greater trochanter
Gluteus minimus: outer surface of the ilium; inserts greater trochanter
Piriformis: ventral sacrum, greater sciatic foramen and superior greater trochanter
Gemellus superior: Spine of ischium and middle part of medial aspect of greater trochanter of femur.
Gemellus Inferior: Upper border of ischial tuberosity and middle part of medial aspect of greater trochanter of femur.
Obturator Internus: Inner surface of obturator membrane and rim of pubis and ischium bordering membrane and middle part of medial aspect of greater trochanter of femur.
Obturator Externus: Outer obturator membrane, rim of pubis and ischium to trochanteric fossa on medial surface of greater trochanter.
Quadratus Femoris: Lateral border of ischial tuberosity and quadrate tubercle of femur.
Actions:
Gluteus Maximus: Hip extension (powerful); external rotation of femur; raises trunk when lower limb is fixed; abduction (upper fibers).

Gluteus Medius: Abduction of femur; internal rotation of femur (anterior fibers); external rotation of femur(posterior fibers); stabilizes pelvis when contralateral foot is off the ground (gait).
Gluteus Minimus: Abduction of femur; internal rotation of femur (anterior fibers); depresses hip when contralateral foot is off the ground (gait).
Lateral rotators: External rotation of femur. Stabilizes the legs while walking and works in tandem with the internal rotators to keep the legs and knees tracking.

The client is prone with feet supported on bolster.

The hip being treated should be put in external rotation and flexion to put excessively tight muscles on slack.

1. Using the concepts of Muscle Swimming, we begin by warming the tissues. The external rotators of the hip (piriformis, gemelli , obdurators & quadratas femoris) are deep to the gluteal group. Warming of the superficial layer of muscles will automatically include the "deep 6". Find the greater trochanter and think of it like the hub of a wheel with all of the gluteal muscles and external rotators attaching to it and then fanning out to attachment sights from tip of tail bone & ischial tuberosity bone almost to the ASIS. Grasping, lifting and kneading the muscles is a good warm-up.

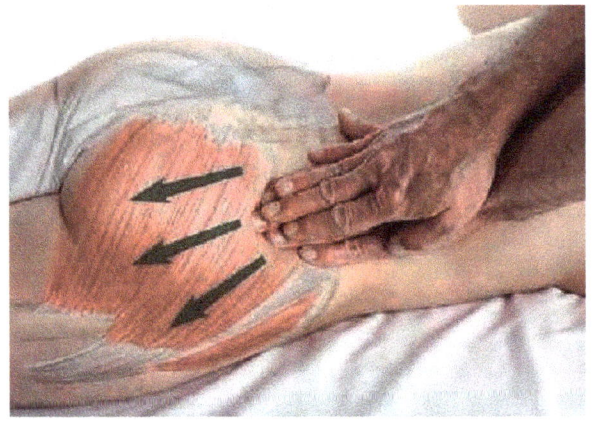
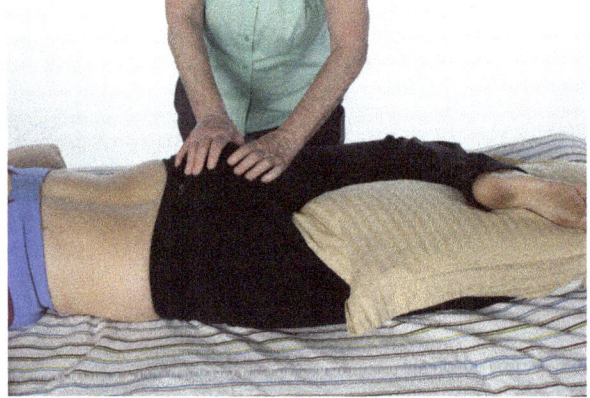

2. Pin and Rock to promote fascial melting: Gently pin the muscles with multiple fingers for a broad, dispersed pressure with one hand and add a slow rhythmic rocking of the pelvis with your other hand.

Right: Pin and Rock

3. Pin and Move: Use more precise pressure such as thumbs, elbows or a tool and revisit any acutely sensitive trigger points. Apply static pressure and have the client fire the muscle by internally and externally rotating the thigh, pelvic tilts or any movement your client thinks would be helpful. Pay special attention to where gluteus maximus connects with IT band. Precise work at lower attachments of gluteus maximus helps to correct this muscle's tendency to misalign the band causing patella tracking issues. Creating left/right balance and relaxing the fibrous attachments of gluteus maximus at the sacrum can be helpful in relieving sacroiliac issues.

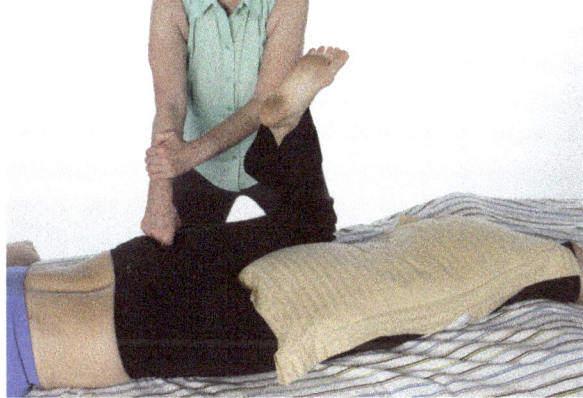
Client doing active internal/external rotation of thigh.

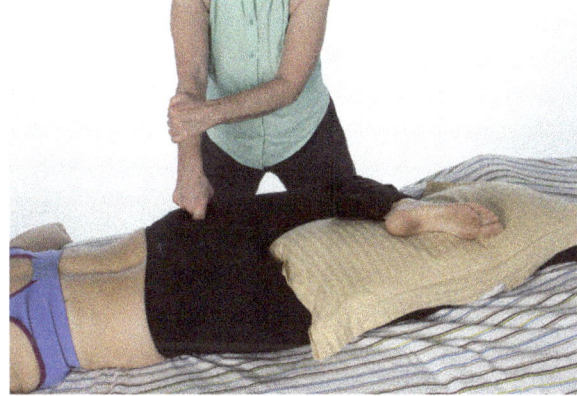
Client doing anterior tilt of pelvis.

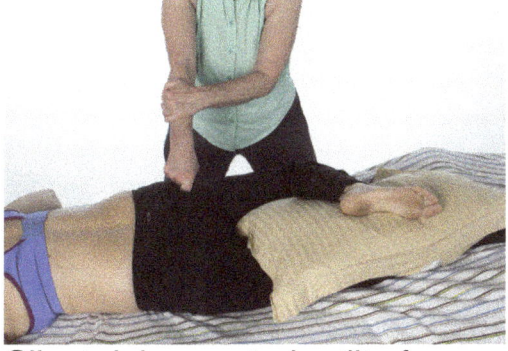
Client doing posterior tilt of pelvis.

Piriformis stretch

Client is supine.

Step 1: Have the client place the ankle of the leg to be stretched on top of the opposite thigh so that the leg to be stretched is externally rotated. (The piriformis becomes an internal rotator when the femur is flexed and abducted and the lower leg crosses the midline. This is why we externally rotate the thigh to stretch the piriformis.)

Step 2: Ask the client to lift the opposite foot off the table, which they can place on your thigh (as shown in photo A) or shoulder (photo B), or a bolster depending on the degree of thigh flexion needed. The degree of thigh flexion of the opposite leg determines the intensity of the piriformis stretch. Ask your client exactly where they feel the stretch. If they only feel it in the hip flexors, increase the amount of thigh flexion of the opposite leg.

Step 3: Increase the degree of external rotation by pulling the client's knee toward you and pushing her ankle away from you.

Note: If you are working with a client who has been suffering from severe piriformis syndrome, be careful with this stretch. Wait until you have worked with the client several times before performing this stretch, and then proceed with caution.

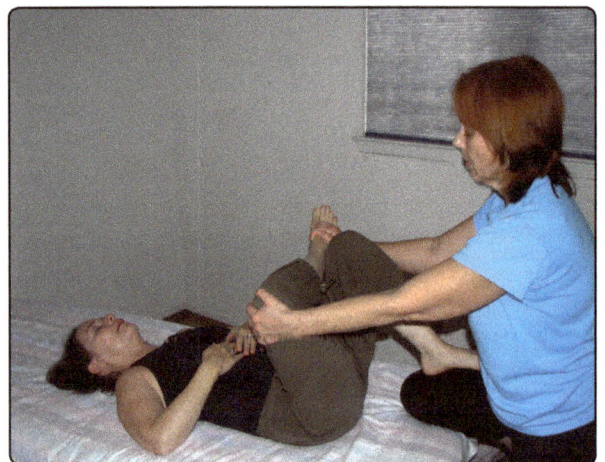

Photo A

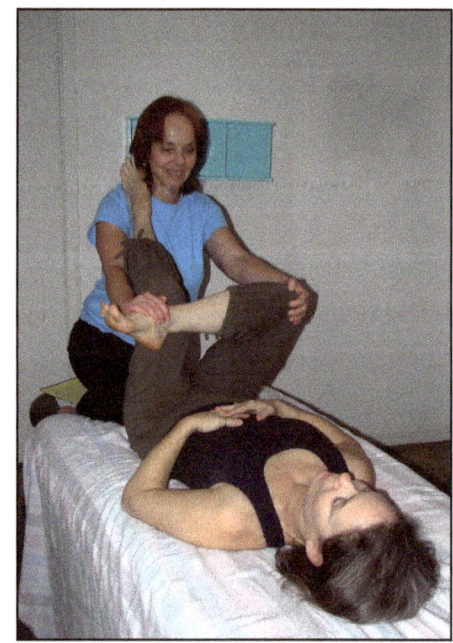

Photo B

Muscle Swimming Techniques for quadratus lumborum

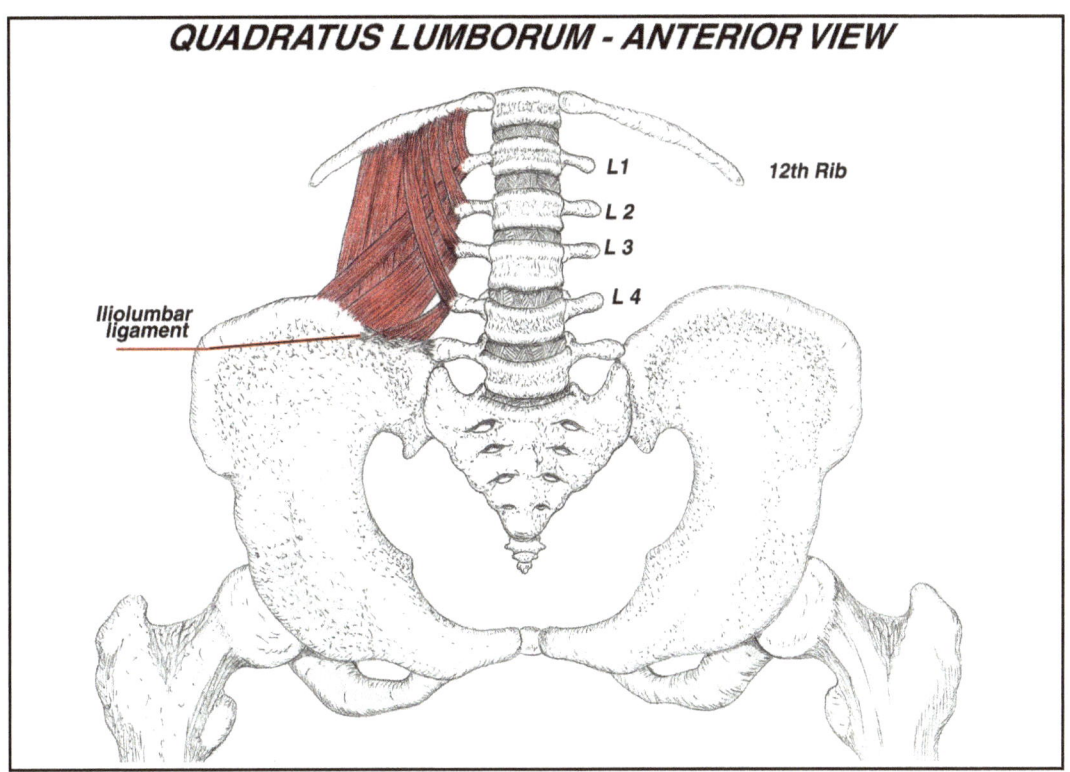

Attachments: (Above) 12th rib and lumbar vertebrae 1-4; (below) ilium and iliolumbar ligament.

Actions: Lateral flexion of the spine; elevation of the ipsilateral ilium (hip hiking); contributes to extension of the spine; stabilizes the 12th rib during inhalation and forced exhalation; plays a significant role in maintaining upright posture. Part of the lateral sling (Gmed, adductors, contralateral QL.). QL tends to be overly-facilitated while the contralateral Gmed tends to be underly-facilitated.

Note: the high-illium QL will be overly-facilitated and the opposite QL will tend to be underly-facilitated. Stretch the high side and strengthen the opposite side.

The side-lying position offers the most advantages for precise deep tissue work on the quadratus lumborum. This position allows us to work the complex fiber arrangement of the QL with more accuracy. In addition, there are more movement options available so we can Muscle Swim through the layers of the sturdy quadratus lumborum. Place a small hand towel under the client's waist — this creates more room for deep tissue work. If possible, place the client's top arm behind her head on the table which elevates the rib cage, again allowing more space for you to work.

Find the iliac crest and the 12th rib, then place your fingers halfway between those bony landmarks. Move your fingers about 1/4 to 1/2 inch posterior and gently press toward the table. You will be on the most lateral layer of the QL. Have your client hike her hip to verify your position. You should feel the robust QL shorten under your fingers. Keep in mind you should be pressing deep to the erector spinae.

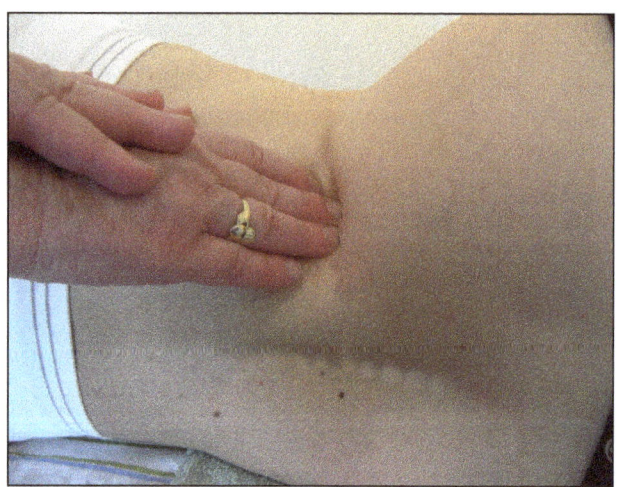

STEP 1: Warm the tissue with gliding stokes which include the thoraco-lumbar fascia.

STEP 2:
A. We'll use the Pin and Rock technique as our way of preparing the QL for deeper work.

Place two or three fingers of your uphill hand on the belly of the QL using gentle pressure. Place your downhill hand on your client's hip. Maintain the moderate pressure on the QL as you slowly rock your client's hips forward and back. The hand on the QL is still, the working hand is the rocking hand. Instruct your client to breathe deeply. Do this until you feel the QL begin to soften.

B. After this central part of the quadratus lumborum softens, angle your fingers to the iliac crest and continue this Pin and Rock technique. Once you feel that section soften, angle your fingers to the 12th rib and continue this technique. Since we're working in a small area, angling the fingers usually suffices to connect with these attachments.

C. Continue with this gentle fascial melting on the deeper layers of the QL at its medial attachments on L1-4.

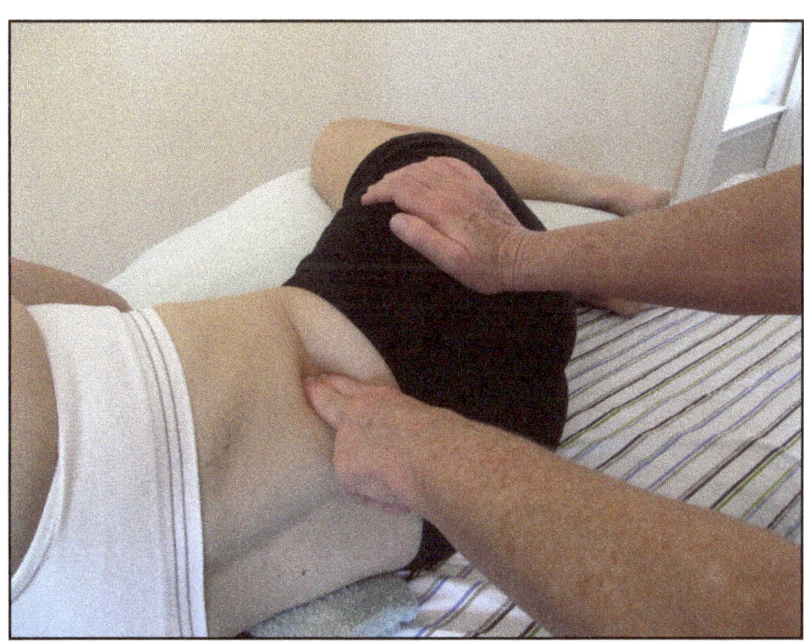

STEP 3: Once the tissue is warm and receptive, it's time to release knots, adhesions, and trigger points with our *Pin and Move* technique. When you feel a knot, adhesion, or trigger point, gently pin the area while the client does active movement.

A technique that's especially useful for an upslipped SIJ, high ilium and anteriorly rotated pelvis is one I call "Running Man". This allows the illium to move inferiorly and the ishium to move anteriorly.

Instructions for Running Man

1. Ask the client to slowly slide the top leg towards the chest, keeping the entire leg in contact with the table. The thigh does not need to come into full flexion. Whatever the client can do without straining is fine. The bottom leg should be comfortable with a small degree of flexion at the thigh and knee.

2. Have her slowly slide the top leg into extension

3. Lift that leg about one inch above the bottom leg and place it behind the bottom leg.

4. Repeat the above steps 3-5 times while working the tissue.

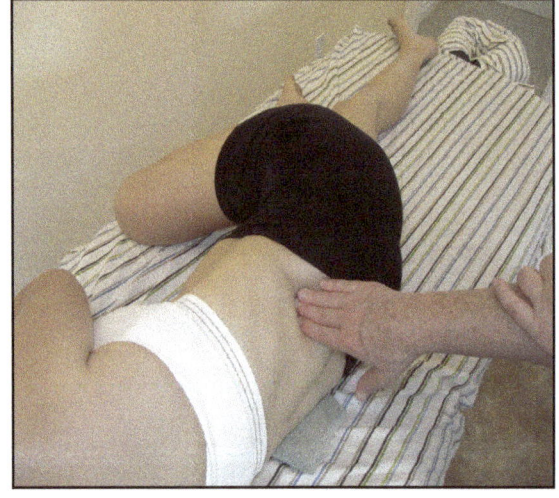

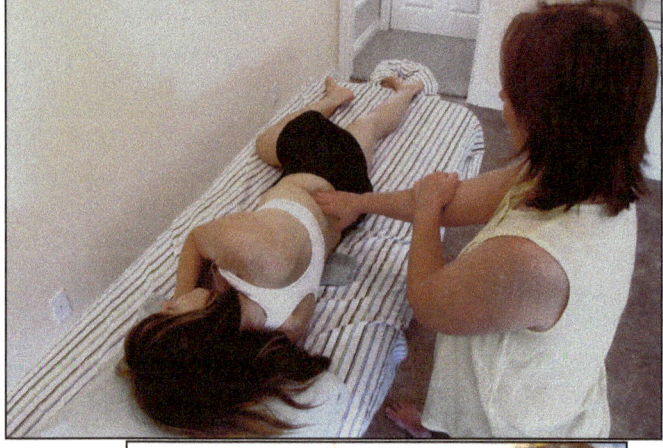

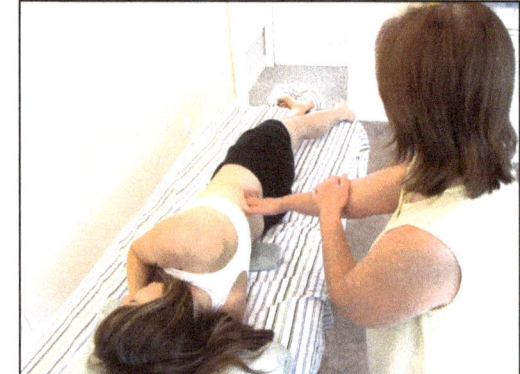

Step One above left: client flexing her thigh

Step Two above right: Client extending her thigh

Step Three right: Placing her thigh behind the bottom leg

Quadratus lumborum stretch

Stretch the **high** ilium/short QL side. Client is side-lying on the side opposite to be stretched and moves her body to the edge of the table. Guide the top leg to hang off the edge of the table. The knee needs to clear the table; sometimes it takes a bit of trial and error to achieve this while maintaining the client's alignment. If you're having trouble getting the knee to clear the table, ask her to scoot her upper body away from you and her rear end towards you. Stabilize the pelvis with your body to prevent rotation or over-arching of the lower back. A towel under the client's waist can help with positioning and increase the stretch. To use a PNF strategy (agonist-contract), have the client push the leg up toward the ceiling (abduction) to engage/shorten the QL, with no more than 20% effort. Client holds the contraction for 8-10 seconds. Therapist then feels if the tissue can stretch farther. Repeat the PNF two more times. PNF techniques are especially good for re-educating the stretch reflex and reducing its signaling on tissue that has an especially short resting length.

Step 1: Gently press down on the femur (less intense) or the calf (more intense) of the leg being stretched with your downhill hand. The client's upper arm must be above the ribs, reaching up towards her head. With your uphill hand traction the iliac crest away from the ribs. Hold for 15-30 seconds.

Step 2: Move your upper hand to the rib case and traction it away from the pelvis, while maintaining the pressure on the femur or calf. Hold for 15-30 seconds.

Step 3: To come out of the stretch, lift the leg back onto the table, so the client does not engage the muscle.

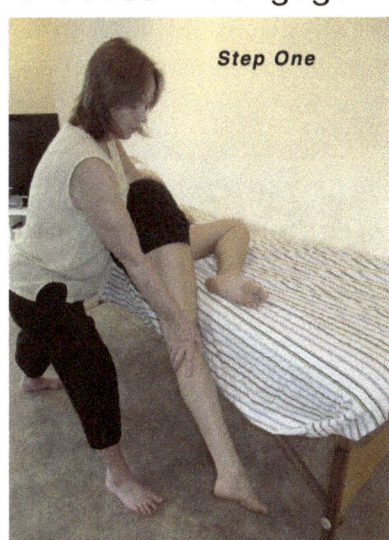
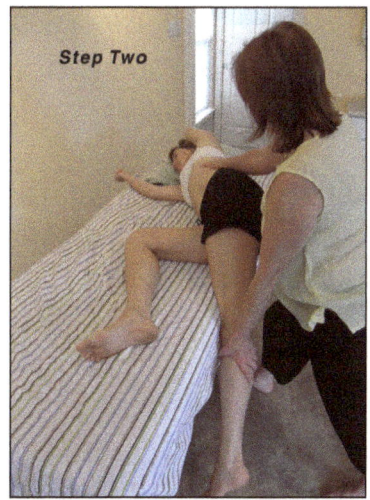

Muscle Swimming Techniques for Multifidus

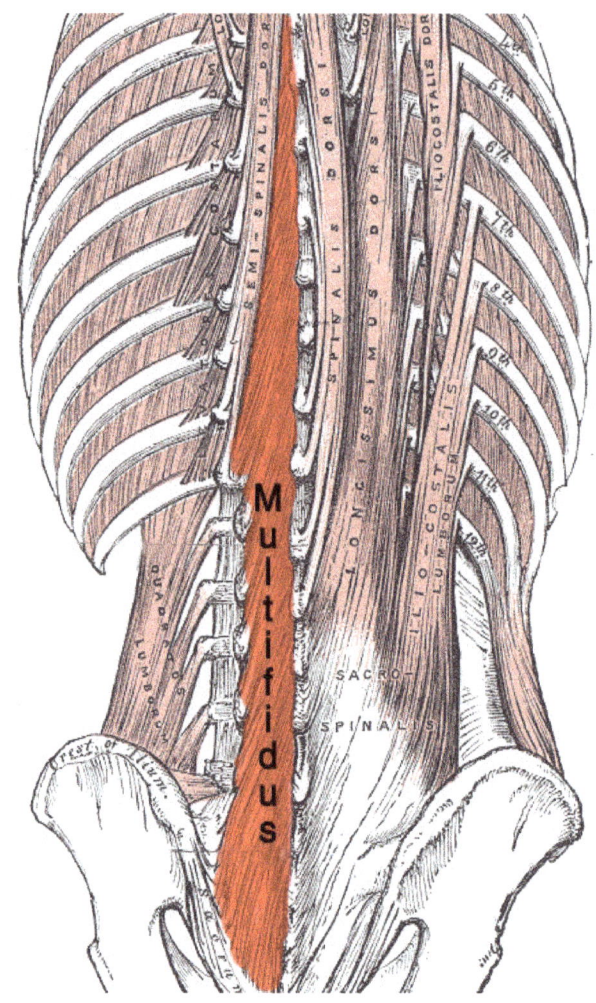

Attachments: : From the posterior surface of the sacrum, iliac crest and the transverse processes of all lumbar, thoracic vertebrae and articular processes of cervical 4-7. These muscles traverse 2-4 vertebrae and attach superiorly to the spinous processes of all vertebrae apart from the atlas.

Actions: Unilaterally – ipsilateral flexion and contralateral rotation. Bilaterally – spinal extension and stabilization. Part of the inner core unit that assists in stabilizing the SI joint.

The client is prone. A small towel or flat pillow may be placed under the belly to correct an anterior rotation of the pelvis.

STEP 1: Using the concepts of Muscle Swimming, we begin by warming the tissues with minimal lubricant. Use a superior to inferior gliding movement.

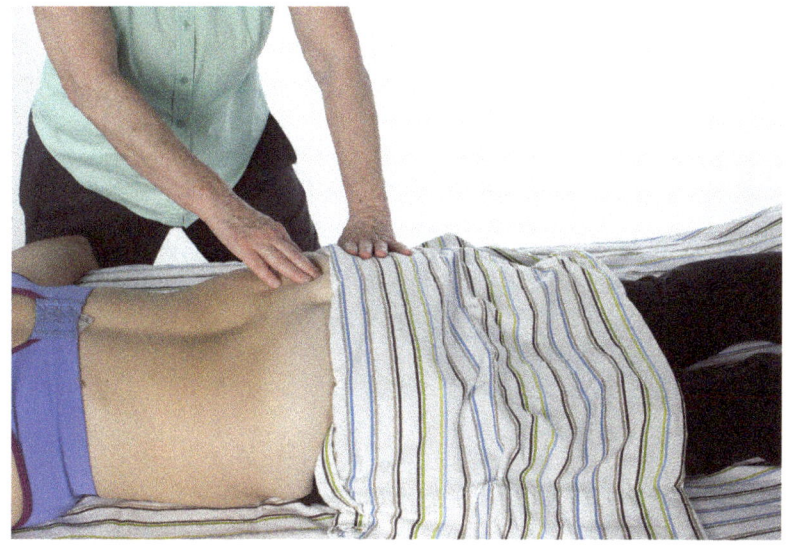

STEP 2: Pin and Rock to promote facial melting: Gently pin the sacral multifidi with multiple fingers for a broad, dispersed pressure with one hand and add a slow rhythmic rocking of either the femur or pelvis with your other hand. Pin and Rock can be done at any point in this protocol.

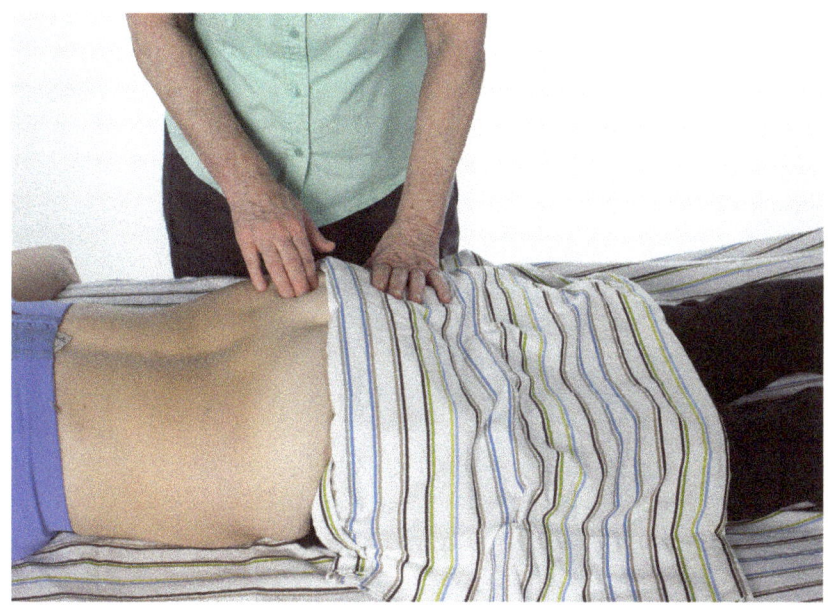

STEP 3: Pin and Move: Using more precise pressure with thumbs, elbows or a tool release any acutely sensitive trigger points and fascial adhesions. Apply static pressure and have the client fire the muscle using active movement by:
a.   Pelvic tilts
b.   Spinal extensions
c.   Any movement your client thinks would be helpful

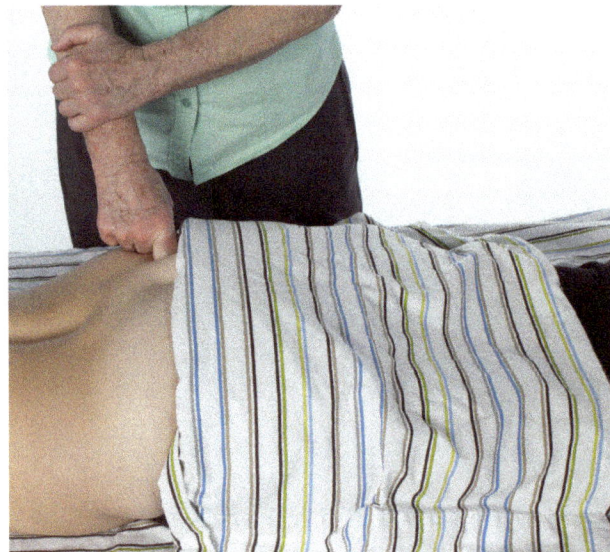

Above: Client performing anterior pelvic tilts

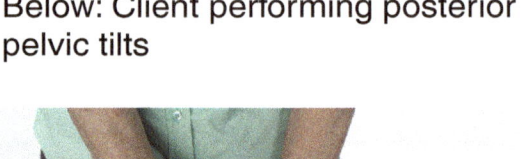

Below: Client performing posterior pelvic tilts

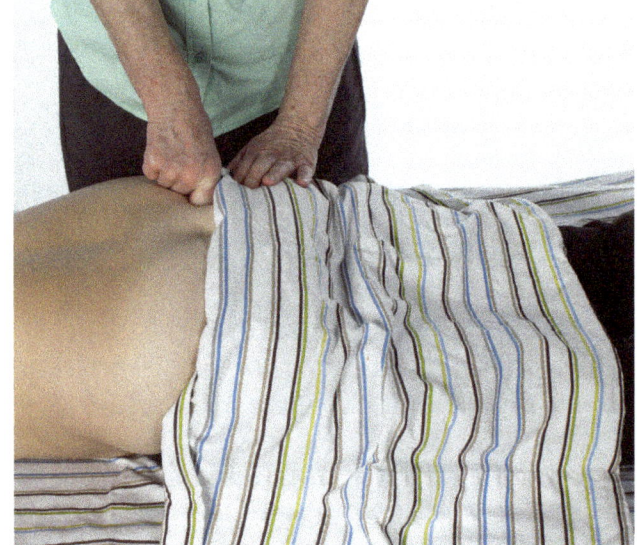

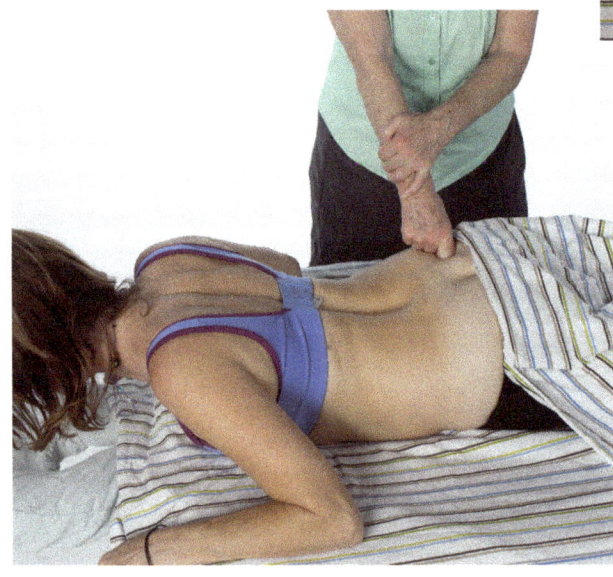

Left: Client performing spinal extension

Muscle Swimming techniques for hamstrings

The Hamstring Group

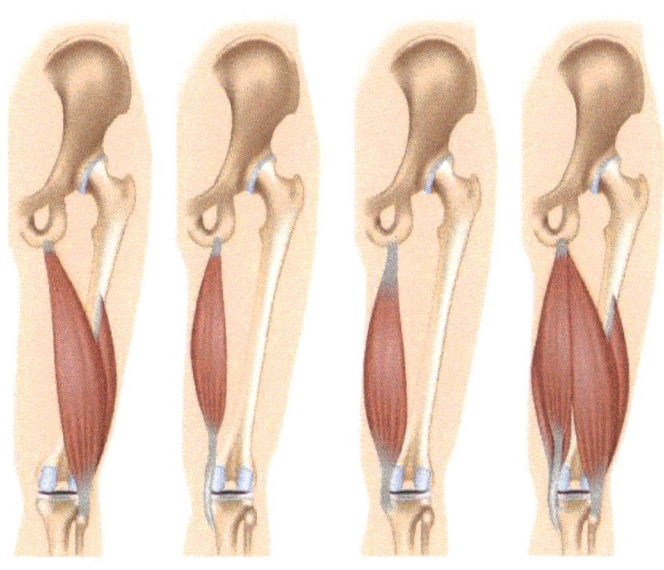

Biceps femoris   Semitendinosus   Semimembranosus

Heads
1. Biceps femoris- long head
2. Biceps femoris- short head
3. Semitendinosus
4. Semimembranosus

Attachments: Superior - Ischial tuberosity (all); Linea aspera of femur (short head of biceps femoris). The long head of biceps femoris blends with the sacrotuberous ligament. Inferior - lateral and medial condyles of tibia; fibular head.

Actions: flexion of the knee, extension of thigh, assists in stabilizing sacrum (example - during forward flexion of the spine, fibers of the long head of biceps femoris restrain the sacrum).

The client is prone. Place a pillow under the anterior calf of leg to be treated to slack the muscle.

Step 1: Using the concepts of Muscle Swimming, we begin by warming the tissues with minimal lubricant. Some options for warming the tissue are compressions or grasping, lifting and kneading the muscles.

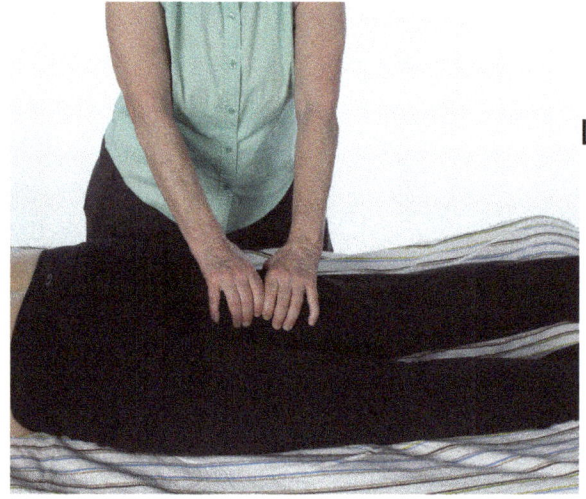

Left: Warming the hamstrings

Step 2: Pin and Rock to promote facial melting: Gently pin the hamstrings with multiple fingers for a broad, dispersed pressure with one hand and add a slow rhythmic rocking of either the femur or pelvis with your other hand.

Step 3: Fascial work: If there is an anteriorly tilted pelvis on the side being treated, the hamstrings are eccentrically overloaded or locked-long. The direction of your myofascial work should be superior to inferior and side to side (think of an S curve) to encourage shortening and restoring normal resting length (Photo below). If there's a posterior tilt the hamstrings are locked-short. Use the same S curve but direct your strokes inferior to superior.

Use a firm yet gentle, sustained pressure, moving slowly through the layers of tissue to assess and release adhesions and thickenings. When you feel a thickened or congested area, or when your fingers stop, unable to drag freely over the tissue, maintain a gentle direct pressure, meeting and melting this barrier, for about 30 seconds to one minute.

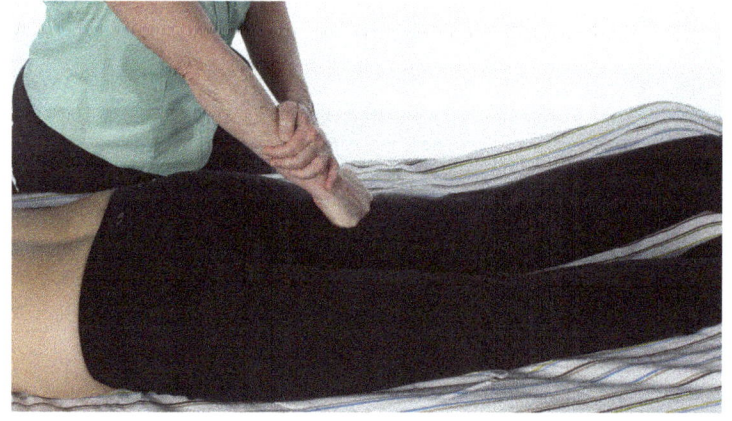

Step 4: Pin and Move. Using more precise pressure with thumbs, elbows or a tool release any acutely sensitive trigger points and fascial adhesions. Apply static pressure and have the client fire the muscle using active movement by:
a. Flexion and extension of knee
b. Thigh extension
c. Pelvic tilts
d. Any movement your client thinks would be helpful

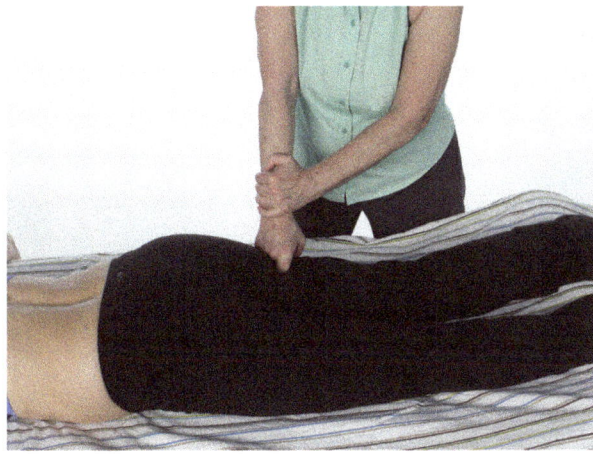

Left: Client performing anterior pelvic tilts

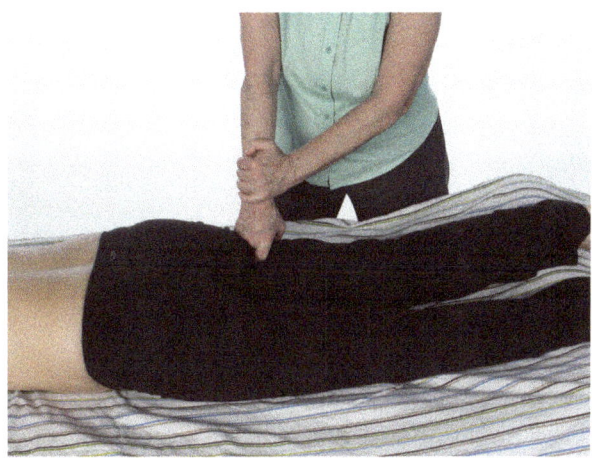

Right: Client performing posterior pelvic tilts

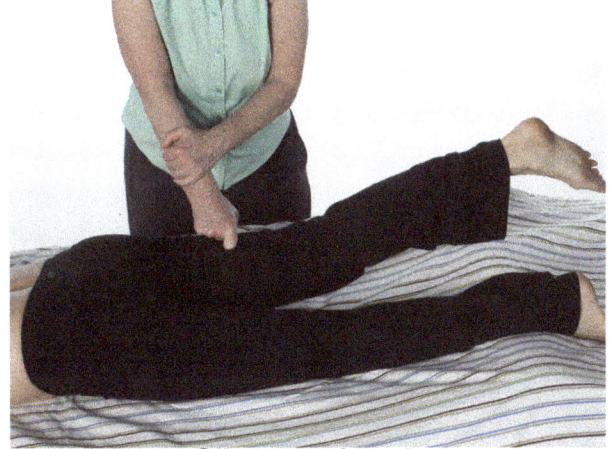

Above: Client performing thigh extensions

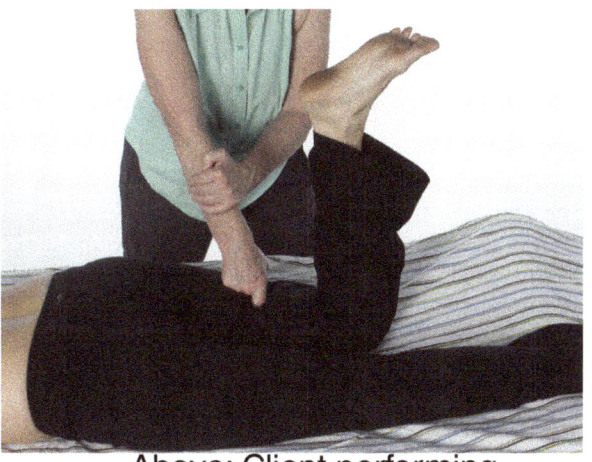

Above: Client performing knee flexion and extension

Check List

Assessment Tests:

1A. Standing test for high ilium: R____ L____ _____

1B. Seated Test for high ilium: R____ L____ _____

2. Test for pelvic tilt: R____ L____ _____

3. Test for upslipped innominate: R____ L____ _____

4. Test for leg length difference (medial malleoli):
   Supine: R____ L____ _____
   Seated: R____ L____ _____

5. Test for Pubic symphysis: R____ L____ _____

6. Test for deep sulcus (apex shift): R____ L____ _____

Corrections:

1. Correction for high ilium: _____

2. Correction for rotation (tilt): _____

3. Correction for upslip: _____

4. Correction for pubic symphysis: _____

5. Correction for deep sulcus: _____

References And Suggested Reading

Chaitow, L. Naturopathic Physical Medicine: Theory and Practice for Manual Therapists. Edinburgh: Churchill Livingstone/Elsevier. 2008
Chaitow, L., & DeLany, J. Clinical application of neuromuscular techniques. Edinburgh: Churchill Livingstone. 2011
Chaitow, L., Franke, H., & Chaitow, L. Muscle energy techniques. Edinburgh: Churchill Livingstone/Elsevier. 2013
Chaitow, Leon, ND, DO. Positional Release Techniques: What are the Mechanisms? Massage Today. January 2016, Volume 16, Issue 01
Chaitow, Leon: The Body's Load-Sharing Hub: The Thoracolumbar Fascia. Massage Today. January 2015. Vol. 15, Issue 01.
Dalton, Eric. Low back, Piriformis and SI joint pain. Massage Today. May 2007
Dalton, Eric. Human Silly Putty. Massage Today. July 2011.
Honig, Peggi. A Case Report of the Treatment of Piriformis Syndrome. Massage Today. January 2007.
Gibbons, John. Muscle energy techniques: A practical guide for physical therapists. Chichester, Eng.: Lotus Pub. 2013
Gibbons, John. Functional Anatomy of the Pelvis and Sacroiliac Joint. Chichester, Eng.: Lotus Pub. 2017.
Gibbons, John. Glutes and the Muscle energy techniques to address them. Massage and Bodywork. July/August 2015
Heller, Marc, DC. Ilio-Sacral Diagnosis and Treatment, Part One. Dynamic Chiropractic. Volume 21. Issue 3. January 2003.
Heller, Marc, DC. Ilio-Sacral Diagnosis and Treatment, Part Two. Dynamic Chiropractic. Volume 21. Issue 6. March 2003.
Jain S. et al TOG. Symphysis pubis dysfunction: a practical approach to management". July 2006
Joseph, Leonard, et. al. Patterns of changes in local and global muscle thickness among individuals with sacroiliac joint dysfunction. Hong Kong Physiotherapy Journal. June 2105
Kapandji, A. I. Physiology of the joints: Volume 3: The spinal cord, pelvic girdle and head. 2008
Kurnik, Joseph, DC. Hamstring Injuries Resulting from Sacroiliac Dysfunction. Dynamic Chiropractic. April 3, 2000, Vol. 18, Issue 08
Learman, KE. Sacroiliac Joint as a Source of Pain: Diagnosis and Management. Manual Therapy for Musculoskeletal Pain Syndromes: An Evidence- and Clinical-Informed Approach. Elsevier Health Science. 2015
Lowe, Whitney. . Orthopedic assessment in massage therapy. Sisters, Or.: Daviau Scott. 2006.
Lowe, Whitney. Exploring the Anterior Pelvic Tilt. Massage Today: July, 2014, Vol. 14, Issue 07
Luchau, Til. Working with the Lumbars: The Thoracolumbar Fascia. Massage and Bodywork. September/October 2014

Luchau, Til. Advanced Myofascial Techniques: Shoulder, Pelvis, Leg and Foot, Volume 1. Handspring Publishing. 2014.

Muscolino, Joseph, DC. Science and Technique: Deliver More Effective Bodywork. Massage and Bodywork Quarterly. March/April 2016.

Rachel, Matthew, et al. A Study to Compare the effectiveness of MET and Joint Mobilization along with Conventional Physiotherapy in the Management of SI Joint Dysfunction. Indian Journal of Physiotherapy and Occupational Therapy. June 2015.

Rausbaum, Ralph et al. Clinical Spine Surgery Sacroiliac Joint Pain and its treatment. March 2016

Roberts, Debbie. Learning a Hands-Fee Solution to Fix SI Dysfunction. Massage Today; December, 2014, Vol. 14, Issue 12

Sacks, Oliver: A Leg to Stand On; HarperCollins; 1984.

Schamberger, Wolf. 2013. The Malalignment Syndrome: diagnosis and treatment of common pelvic and back pain. 2nd Edition. Churchilhill Livingstone, Elsever

Sweigard, Lulu. Human Movement Potential - Its Ideokinetic Facilitation, Harper and Row.1974

Travell, Janet & Simons, David. Myofascial Pain and Dysfunction: The Trigger Point Manual, William and Wilkens. 1992

Index

A
Adaptation 9
Anterior Pelvic Rotation Correction 36, 37
Assessment Tests 17

C
Check List 61
Core Stability 5
Corrections 31

F
Force closure 13
Form closure 13

G
Gender Difference 8
Gluteal group and external rotators of the hip 46

H
Hamstrings 58
High Iliac Crest Correction 34

L
Left on Left rotation 11
Ligaments and the SIJ 14

M
Multifidus 55
Muscle Energy Techniques 32
Muscles and the SIJ 15
Myofascial sling systems 13

N
Nutation and Counter-nutation 10

P
Pelvic Girdle Anatomy 6
Piriformis muscle 16
Piriformis stretch 49
PNF 54
Posterior oblique sling 15
Principles of Muscle Swimming 42, 45
Pubic Symphysis Correction 39

Q
Quadratus lumborum 50, 55

R
References And Suggested Reading 62
Right on Right rotation 11

S
Sacral Torsion 11
Sacral Torsion Correction 40
Sacroiliac Upslip Corrrection 38
Self-locking mechanism of the SI joint 13

T
Test for anterior or posterior rotation 21
Test for high Iliac crest 18
Test for leg length difference (medial malleoli) 25
Test for Pubic Symphysis 27
Test for Sacral Torsion
Test for upslipped innominate 23

Peggy Lamb, MA, LMT, BCTMB will tell you she is a massage therapist. She is a massage therapist, but she is so much more than that. When Peggy confronts a problem, she doesn't just solve the problem for herself. She will solve the problem for others, and try to insure that the problem isn't a problem for all her clients. When she tore a rotator cuff, she learned about shoulders, about how they move, how the function, and how they function well. Not only did she completely recover from her injury, she wrote a book "Releasing the Rotator Cuff" so other massage therapists can help their clients with shoulder injuries. When faced with a back injury, Peggy worked to recover from that, and recover she did. Not content to just overcome her own injury, she wrote another book "The Core of the Matter: Releasing the Iliopsoas and Quadratus Lumborum", with content 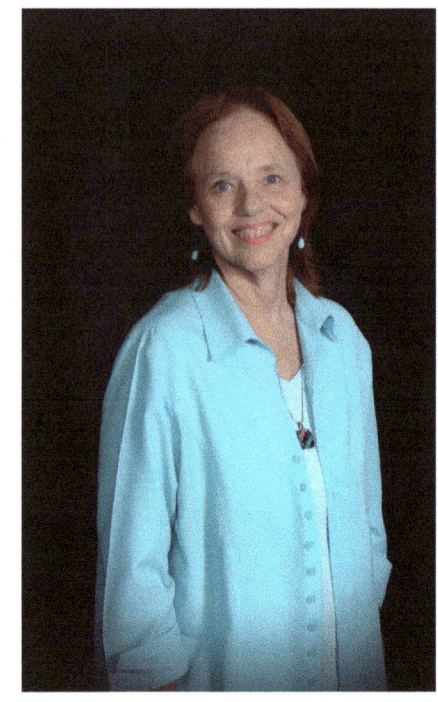 geared to help others, and other massage therapists, with back problems. Peggy doesn't just fix issues that come up in her life, but she fixes those issues for others. Peggy Lamb is not just a massage therapist, she is an author of three books, a creator of 3 DVD instructional sets, a teacher of massage therapist, a leader in her field. All of this comes from one feeling.….the desire to touch, to heal, and to be touched.

Peggy has practiced massage since 1986 and is nationally certified. She currently owns a private massage and movement therapy business, where she practices when she's not teaching. Peggy received her initial training at the New Mexico Academy of Massage and Advanced Healing Arts in Santa Fe, New Mexico, and at Wellness Skills, Inc., in Dallas, Texas. She taught Clinical Anatomy and Physiology, Trigger Point therapy, Designing a Treatment Strategy and Swedish technique at Wellness Skills, Inc., in Dallas and at Texas Healing Arts Institute in Austin. Peggy has taught for Vyne Education for over ten years.

In addition to her extensive training in massage therapy, Peggy holds a master's degree in Dance from American University in Washington, D.C. She has volunteered for 10 years with "Truth be Told", teaching creative movement and writing to incarcerated women. Peggy brings her eclectic and extensive background into her teaching for an interesting, enjoyable and enlightening learning experience. When she's not working, Peggy can be found dancing, swimming in Austin's Barton Springs, hiking or even dog sledding.

www.ingramcontent.com/pod-product-compliance
Lightning Source LLC
Chambersburg PA
CBHW041344020526
44112CB00062B/2953